Understanding the Changing Brain

A Positive Approach to Dementia Care

Understanding the Changing Brain

Move from Surviving to Thriving with Teepa Snow's Tips and Insights

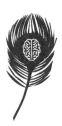

Teepa Snow, MS, OTR/L, FAOTA

Founder of Positive Approach to Care

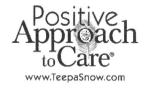

www.TeepaSnow.com

Published by Positive Approach, LLC
Efland, NC

ISBN: 978-1-7359373-4-2 - Paperback
eISBN: 978-1-7359373-5-9 - eBook

Library of Congress Control Number:

Printed in the United States of America   072621

⊗This paper meets the requirements of ANSI/NISO Z39.48-1992 (Permanence of Paper)

We would like to celebrate and dedicate this book to those advocates and individuals who are making amazing strides by choosing to do it differently, and **live life fully, while living with dementia.**

I'm trying not to get exasperated, but this is really hard. I don't like what's happening—it's really tough to see these changes and not know what to do.

-Frustrated Family Member

I've heard a lot of different things about dementia. It's hard to know what to believe. Sometimes people pretend nothing has changed, while I notice that a lot of things are different now.

-Curious and Concerned

Table of Contents

Introduction to *A Positive Approach to Dementia Care* Book Series

By Debi Tyler Newsom and Dan Bulgarelli

If you are curious about dementia, living with dementia, caring for someone with dementia, or wanting to support a friend or family member on this journey, this book series is for you. Throughout her professional career, Teepa Snow has worked to help people understand what dementia is, how it affects a person's life, and what can be done to maintain a meaningful life filled with joy. She has presented to thousands of audiences worldwide and written articles for everyone to see. We have organized several of these articles into books that we think will be helpful to you, addressing the common questions that come up related to loving and caring for a person who is experiencing brain change.

When we think about the brain, we may consider it a single unit. The truth is, there are many different parts of the brain that are all working at the same time to help us learn from and navigate our lives. Each part of the brain is responsible for receiving, sending, and/or analyzing the data received through our senses, combining that with prior knowledge of the situation, and choosing what to do next. All of this is constantly happening in a fraction of a second. The brain is a truly marvelous thing! We are continually learning more about brain function as well as brain change related to dementia.

This book explains what dementia is, and what changes a person living with dementia can experience, and provides some helpful tips for those who provide care and support. Future books in the series will include topics such as personal care and activities of daily living, care for the caregiver, supporting and informing others, environmental considerations, and finding purpose and joy in the daily routine.

Our hope is that this book series will help you use Teepa's insight about the human brain and dementia to move beyond just getting by and surviving this journey, to actually thriving and finding moments of joy.

There are some words and phrases in this book you might not be familiar with, so we wanted to provide a brief introduction. These word choices are referred to as PAC Language (Positive Approach to Care = PAC).

1. Care Partner – While more people are familiar with the term **caregiver**, we prefer to say **care partner**. The

reason for this subtle shift is the basis of our philosophy – that we are supporting a person living with dementia – we are helping them do things or doing things *with* them, we don't do things *to* them. The relationship comes first, we are in this together, we are partners. We do what we do, <u>ultimately</u>, with their permission, in some form or fashion.

2. GEMS° State – You will see references to the GEMS State Model or possibly a particular GEMS State that a person may be experiencing at that moment. There are six different GEMS States – Sapphire, Diamond, Emerald, Amber, Ruby, and Pearl. Teepa created the GEMS State Model to help people better understand retained abilities and areas where support may be needed throughout the progression of dementia, based on the Allen Cognitive Scale. The reason she created a new model is that most scales are based on a numerical system, and numbers have an inherent value. Would you rather have 1 cookie or 3? Would you rather be in 1st place or 6th? When we look at people living with dementia as being in various GEMS States, we begin to see them as individuals with characteristics, and each is precious, unique, and with value. They are different, yes, but one is not inherently better than another. Most importantly, given the right care and setting, they can all shine.

3. Person or People Living with Dementia (PLwD) –

The emphasis is on the **person first**, rather than putting the focus on the disease. Dementia isn't what defines a person and it isn't a choice. Instead, it is a condition that the person, and those around them, are learning to live with and constantly adapt to.

4. Alzheimer's vs. Alzheimers vs. Alzheimer – this subtle shift in spelling and punctuation is indicative of the commonality of the term. Many of us have moved to stating it as Alzheimer disease or Alzheimers Disease, but it is still common to see Alzheimer's. All of these spelling variations refer to the same neuro-degenerative brain condition. In this book, anything we write will not have the apostrophe. When you see the apostrophe, we are quoting someone else or using the name of an organization that uses the apostrophe.

5. Alzheimers vs. Dementia – while the term Alzheimers is often used in place of dementia, they are not equal. Alzheimers is one subset of dementia. As of the writing of this book, there are over 120 known types, forms, and causes of dementia. If we know that someone is living with Alzheimers, we know that they are living with dementia. On the other hand, if someone is living with dementia, it may be Alzheimers, Lewy Body Dementia, Vascular Dementia, or one of the other types, forms, or causes.

You may see a few other words or phrases you aren't familiar with. If you'd like to know more, please check out our website: www.teepasnow.com

Scan this code with your smartphone's camera or visit **www.teepasnow.com/moreinfo** on your computer.

Introduction to
Understanding the Changing Brain

Brain Change-What is Dementia All About?

When we talk about dementia, any kind of dementia, we are talking about brain change or brain failure. To be fair, we all experience episodes of brain change even when dementia is not present. Have you ever found yourself to be impatient or short-tempered with someone when you are hungry? What about when you haven't been getting enough sleep or you are under a lot of stress?

The difference between dementia and those examples of brain change, is that with sustenance, sleep, or relaxation our brain will return to normal. With dementia, there is a progression of both chemical and structural change that prevents the brain's return to *normal*. That isn't to say that sustenance, sleep, relaxation – or the lack thereof – doesn't impact the brain of a person living with dementia, it certainly can and does, it is just that the brain can't return to where it was before dementia was present.

Understanding the basics of how the brain works will help us become more aware that with dementia there are changes that cannot be reversed, but at the same time, there are abilities we can maximize to make life more satisfying for all.

As you read this book, and other books in the series, I will do my best to:

1. describe what is changing in the brain
2. help you understand how these changes affect the person and how they experience the world
3. offer skills and things to try that will allow everyone to find more success, more joy, and better relationships.

The last item is probably the most important. It won't do any good to know about the brain changes of dementia if those of us *able* to make changes are unwilling to try new things. A person living with dementia is doing the best they can at any given moment. It is up to us to recognize this and try to figure out how to support them so we can all thrive together.

When you look at the image on the next page, consider how a change or loss in any one of these areas would drastically affect function. This will help you to begin to understand what life is like for a person living with dementia.

Brain Change Affects Function

Occipital Lobe
- Visual data is processed

Parietal Lobe / Frontal Lobe
•• Sensations are processed and action messages are sent to the spinal nerves

Pre-frontal Lobe
- Logic and reason
- Impulse control
- Making choices
- Self-awareness
- Awareness of others
- Initiating, sequencing, finishing

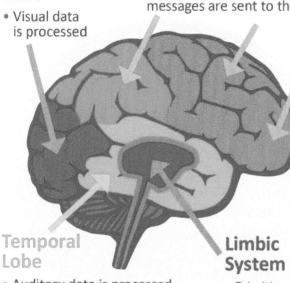

Temporal Lobe
- Auditory data is processed
- Hearing, comprehension, speech production, vocabulary, rhythm related skills

Limbic System
- Primitive brain
- Survival
- Impulses

Graphic 1

CHAPTER 1

It's Not *How*, It's the *Why* that Makes It Work for Me!

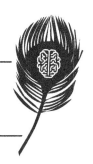

"I don't know how you do it," is probably one of the most common comments I get when I am on the road – when people are reviewing my schedule, or if someone is wondering when I could meet with them and I pull out my phone calendar to try to find a spot.

Here's the thing. It's not the **how** of it. Yeah, that's hard, sometimes grueling, sometimes frustrating, and sometimes requiring incredible flexibility and in-the-moment problem solving beyond what is reasonable. The way I manage to do all of this stuff, is that I get a huge return on investment. No, not financially. Instead, what makes all of this doable is the amazing and remarkable gifts I receive in return. The hugs and tears, the comments, excitement, stories, and the faces of people who are changed. The reports on how they have used that new-found awareness, knowledge, or skill to change the relationships they are in, the work they are doing, or the life they are living. It turns out that in every offering I provide, there is at least one person who is impacted - changed in some way that opens a door or window into another space, another view, another perspective that alters what is happening for them and those around them. How remarkable is that? That is fuel for my spirit and feeds my soul. To know that I help others, and through their work, help beyond my physical reach or visual regard. That is the thing that makes it all possible to do.

As to the how do I do it, well that is a good bit more complicated! The fact of the matter is that *I can't and don't do it on my own, anymore.* Actually, I never did. Dick, my husband of over 40 years, has always been a part of this activity in some fashion. Although, he rarely accompanies me on my crazy journeys, he has managed the banking side of life since the start. There was a time when Dick was still running his business full-time that I was pretty much operating solo. I managed all my travel, booking, billing, services, slideshows, communications, and the other sundry details of being all over the US and Canada, consulting with a senior living company in Georgia, and working for the Eastern NC Chapter of the Alzheimer's Association.

I began to realize that even traveling 250 days a year for my talks and consultations, I couldn't reach as many people as *I* wanted or as often as *they* wanted. One of the messages I try to help everyone working in the world of dementia understand is *you need a team.* It was then that I realized I needed a team as well. I began working with a group in Florida to help get videos of my workshops into DVD format so that people could watch it on their schedule in their home. I wrote a book for the many of us that prefer to read instead of watching something, but I was just scratching the surface. How could I help more people improve their own world of dementia care, one mind at a time? A team!

I have been fortunate to work with some amazing people as part of my team. I won't list them all here because I'm sure I'll forget one, but I hope I have let them all know how much they mean to me and how they have helped me. What I know is that there is no one size fits all when it comes to dementia care; different people need different things. Individuals were asking for more videos. Organizations wanted us to train their staff. Groups wanted us to help develop skills. Dementia isn't only in my home country, the United States, so I was asked to come to Canada, and then the UK, and as of the writing of this book, I have also presented in Poland and Australia with more requests coming in.

With my team growing, we began offering more options based on what people were requesting. We now offer DVDs, streaming options, physical products, books, staff training, certification courses, and…so much more as we learn what people want and need.

One of our most important resources has been our Online

Dementia Journal – which is where most of these articles are pulled from. Each month, Positive Approach to Care puts out a free digital journal with articles and videos; some by me, some by my team, and some created by others in our world that want to share something that has worked for them and they, in turn, want to help others. I encourage you to check it out, sign up, and receive this valuable resource.

So back to the original question: How do I do it? Well, it's a mission. To help change what is currently happening to too many people living with dementia or other forms of brain change and their care providers into something I would want to have happen for me, if I am ever in need of it. To keep my eyes on the prize and my head on track, I often consider these quotes from some of the people I admire most.

You must be the change you wish to see in the world.

Mahatma Gandhi

It is better to light a candle, than curse the darkness.

It is not fair to ask of others what you are not willing to do yourself.

You must do the things you think you cannot do.

I think at a child's birth, if a mother could ask a fairy godmother to endow it with the most useful gift, it would be curiosity.

All by Eleanor Roosevelt

God grant me the serenity to accept the things I cannot change, the courage to change the things I can, and the wisdom to know the difference.

St Francis of Assisi

As for me –

- I am doing my best to promote change for the better through what I do.
- I try to create and offer new possibilities rather than get frustrated with what is not happening or even worse at times, what is.
- I try hard not to ask for what I am not willing to tackle myself.
- I apparently had a super fairy godmother because I am forever curious about what is possible and what comes next.
- That last piece, serenity-courage-wisdom, well, I'm still sorting these out!

PAC Core Values

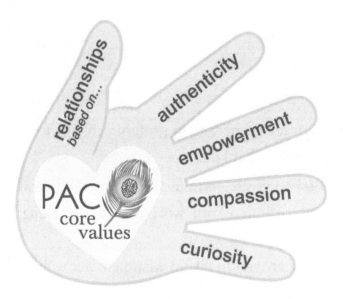

Mission

Use our talents and abilities to develop awareness, spread knowledge, and teach skills to transform what exists into a more positive dementia care culture.

Vision

Positive Approach to Care enhances the life and relationships of those living with brain change by fostering an inclusive universal community.

Graphic 2

CHAPTER 2

Dementia—What's Old, What's New, What's Been Tried, What's True?

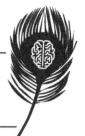

Over the past few years, we have learned a lot more about this thing called *dementia.*

We know now that it is more accurately called *neurodegeneration.* The neurons in the brain are deteriorating and dying.

Scientists have rethought the original theories about causes of one of the major conditions, Alzheimers. There are new thoughts about glial cells, inflammation, brain nutrition, and tau protein malformations being elements that may be triggers for the cascade of events that lead to the beginnings of Alzheimers. Work is being done. Answers are still uncertain.

There are more varied efforts to reduce risk and pause or slow the transition from pre-condition to activation of a condition. Some researchers are aiming toward the idea that perhaps this will be like AIDS. Stop it at HIV, and you can live long and well for many, many years in a high-risk but non-progressive state.

In a very early collaborative publication printed by Aspen Publications in 1988, while I was teaching as part of the Program on Aging at the Medical School at the University of North Carolina, Chapel Hill, I helped to create a *Handbook of Geriatric Practice Essentials*. In this book, I described *dementia* as a big category and *Senile Dementia Alzheimer's Type (SDAT)* as a major form of this thing called dementia when it came to elders. SDAT was designed to replace less friendly and inaccurate terms such as senility and organic brain syndrome (OBS). At the time we thought hardening of the arteries was probably some part of this condition as well.

In 1995, when I was working on a Teaching Nursing Homes project, I began using an umbrella image on my presentations to represent the condition we call *dementia*. Under that early umbrella, I had the overarching term *Alzheimers Disease* with two forms in a huge box below: *Early Onset* and *Normal Onset*. I added another smaller box and called it *Other Dementias*. At the time, the wisdom was that Alzheimers accounted for almost all dementia, with the other types being rare and very unusual. To some extent there was an unspoken belief that getting Alzheimers after age 65 was pretty normal. Therefore, it was referred to as *Normal Onset*. Boy, were they wrong about that!

In 2006, I used an updated umbrella drawing to help people understand the difference between the terms, *Alzheimers* and *dementia*. I was identified as being very unusual at the time for separating out all of the dementias and focusing on the umbrella term, rather than the favorite, but inaccurate word of the day, *Alzheimers.*

I believed *vascular dementia* should be given a bigger and bolder seat at the table, whereas others said it was only a small player. It turns out I was correct! Vascular dementia is probably responsible for roughly 20–30% of neurodegeneration. It is often found in conjunction with Alzheimers or other dementias. It also turns out that of all dementias, it may be one of the first to be slowed or halted with programs that recognize early indicators of problems with brain circulation. If we work hard to keep blood pressure in a lower range at younger ages, blood sugars under control, and focus on heart–healthy brain strategies, perhaps we can change the course or speed of change.

In 2018, Lewy Body Dementia (LBD) became an accepted category for neurodegeneration that is caused by alpha-synuclein protein malformations in brain cells. It was noted that Parkinsons disease was also caused by the same malformed protein, and initial symptoms would typically predict which condition it was. The bad news is that in some cases, both conditions would occur in the same person.

There had also been a change in thinking about how common Lewy Body Dementia was. Lewy Body Dementia is now considered fairly common and when combined with

Parkinsonian-related dementia, may well appear in close to 30% of all cases. In 2017, The **Dementia with Lewy Bodies Consortium** updated the diagnostic criteria for the condition. The U.S. Federal Government now has Research Centers of Excellence to study and better understand the condition and the medical actions that might help diagnose, manage symptoms, or provide care support for people living with Lewy Body Dementia. It is hoped that these efforts will begin to inform medical providers, clinical providers, family members, and people living with Lewy Body Dementia, so that care will improve.

A reasonable outcome might be that fewer incidents of misdiagnosis with mismanagement of care will occur. It might be that there will be a decrease in unnecessary psychiatric or emergency room admissions with better awareness and information. More importantly, perhaps, is that people living with Lewy Body Dementia will be recognized for their retained abilities, their inconsistent symptoms, and their **extremely high risk** of negative impact of many medications or interventions that are used. The risk of mismanagement and mistreatment of common symptoms such as hallucinations, delusional thinking, or sleep disturbances might decrease, and life could be improved.

Since around 2010, our appreciation and understanding of the frontal temporal dementias (FTDs) has also expanded. Appreciating the various types and forms of this condition does matter. It is now generally acknowledged by members of the dementia care culture that frontal temporal dementias are the most common type of young onset dementia. These conditions, in combination, are actually more common than young onset Alzheimers. **The Association for Frontotemporal Degeneration (theAFTD.org)** is a great source of up-to-date information and support for those who are trying to adapt to life with some form of frontal temporal dementia. While there are many forms of this dementia, the Association for FTD has categorized them and included some conditions in a slightly different way than many other systems and sources. Over the next little bit, perhaps we will reach some common ground.

- The National Center for Biotechnology Information (ncbi.nlm.nih.gov) created a test using focused ultrasound with microbubbles for the opening of the blood-brain barrier. The goal is to reduce amyloid-b plaques and tau phosphorylation, improving overall cognitive performance[1].

- Frontal temporal dementias and ALS (amyotrophic lateral sclerosis – Lou Gehrig's disease), it turns out, are related in their genetics, clinical symptoms, and neuropathologies. This fosters a collaborative and

---

[1] Souza RMDCE, da Silva ICS, Delgado ABT, da Silva PHV, Costa VRX. Focused ultrasound and Alzheimer's disease A systematic review. *Dement Neuropsychol.* 2018;12(4):353-359. doi:10.1590/1980-57642018dn12-040003

cross-condition research pathway. What is being learned about ALS may be useful in working to treat at least some forms of FTD and vice versa.

- As for Alzheimers, in December 2017, the **National Institute on Aging (nia.NIH.gov)** created a consortium to enhance research into treating Alzheimers. This consortium connects top-tier researchers and their labs to move efforts in a more organized and integrated fashion. One finding of interest is that gut bacteria and **gut health is tightly connected to brain health**[2], at least for animals. That means that what many of us accepted for quite some time is beginning to be recognized as being true; the blood-brain barrier is not as solid as previously believed, **and** what we eat and how much we eat really does matter for brain health and well-being!

People living with various forms of dementia are becoming active and effective advocates for themselves. Care partners are no longer silent victims and bystanders. They are seeking that which they need to provide better support and care and to break the historic chain of solo caregivers becoming overwhelmed by the enormity of the changes that will need to be

---

[2] Bodogai M, et al. Commensal bacteria contribute to insulin resistance in aging by activating innate B1a cells. *Science Translational Medicine.* 2018 Nov 14;10(467). doi: 10.1126/scitranslmed.aat4271.

navigated. **Dementia Alliance International (DementiaAllianceInternational.org), Dementia Action Alliance (DAAnow.org)**, and other organizations and individuals, are speaking out and providing a new view of life with neurodegeneration. Facebook groups are active and promoting sharing. One group called *Joining the Dots for Dementia* is run by Sarah Ashton, and she is a great resource and information seeker and sharer. There are many more voices speaking out and speaking up!

As you compare the pictures below, you can see that we have updated our umbrella to more accurately reflect what we've learned about the different dementias. Additionally, we have developed new resources, products, and services to meet current needs. During the COVID-19 pandemic, we responded by converting all in-person speaking and training options to virtual learning and support. We have connected with international audiences in Poland, the UK, Australia, and other countries to expand practical and positive care support, awareness, and knowledge with those who are seeking more skill in respectful and effective care provision.

Teepa's Original Umbrella, 1995

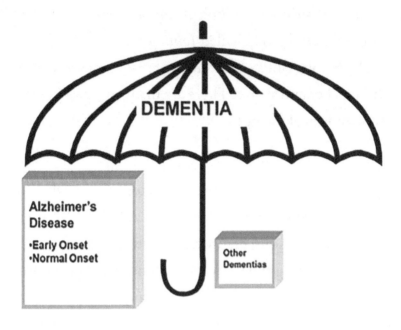

Graphic 3

Teepa's Updated Umbrella, 2019

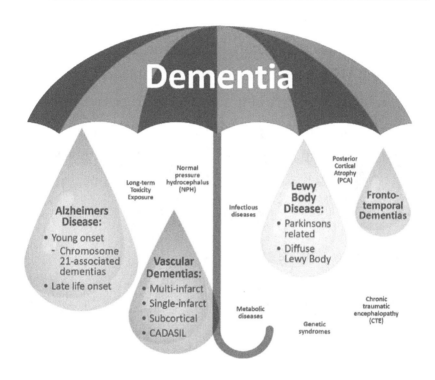

Graphic 4

So, what does all this new information mean for us at Positive Approach to Care®?

It means **we** have more awareness and knowledge ourselves that will help us develop and use skills which promote well-being and positive interactions. It encourages us to continue to ask questions, get curious, build relationships, and stay passionate. We remain committed to building inclusive, informed, and helpful communities where there is support for those living with changing abilities, through words and actions that are respectful and encouraging, as well as accepting and forgiving. This will ensure an environment where all can prosper.

Different Dementias, Different Symptoms

Alzheimers

- Ability to retain new details lost first
- Recent memory worse than old
- Some language problems, mis-speaks or misunderstands
- More impulsive or indecisive
- Makes mistakes about time, place, or situations

Lewy Body

- On/Off symptoms
- Movement problems – falls, hand use, swallowing
- Visual disturbances about animals, people, or children
- Delusional thinking or dreams seem real
- Episodes of inability to move or sudden drops in BP, heart rate, or blood sugar
- Insomnia – sleep disturbances

Vascular

- Abilities are often stable, then there are sudden losses, afterward some recovery
- Symptom combinations are highly variable
- Can have good days and bad days; least predictable
- Judgment and behavior not the same as before
- Emotional and energy shifts can happen quickly

Fronto-temporal

Frontal
(impulse and behavior control changes):

- Says unexpected, rude, mean, odd things
- Apathy – not caring
- Problems with initiation or sequencing
- Dis-inhibited: sex, food, drink, emotions, actions

Temporal
(language change):

- Difficulty with speaking – missing/ changing words
- Rhythm OK, content missing
- Not getting messages

Four Truths About All Dementias:

- At least two parts of the brain are dying
- It keeps changing and getting worse – progressive
- It is not curable or fixable – chronic
- It results in death – terminal

Graphic 5

CHAPTER 3

I Am Who I Was, But I'm Different: Being the ME I Choose to Be

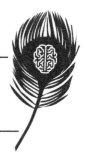

We all have a variety of personas we use in various life situations. We behave differently based on our audience, the environment, and the feedback we receive. Even our appearance will change based on where we are and with whom we are spending time. A person's behavior tends to be quite different while attending a worship service versus having a close friend over to watch a hotly contested ballgame. A key difficulty with dementia is that the person's ability to successfully interpret the environment and select and perform the socially acceptable role is gradually lost. The loss leaves only the private self on view at all times resulting in behaviors that others find irritating and problematic in public situations.

The purpose of this article is four-fold. The primary purpose is to discuss the various selves we use. Second, we will identify how we typically determine which self to show in differing situations. Then we will describe the impact of dementia on one's ability to choose between our different selves. Finally, we will identify strategies that may be helpful in training staff and family in coping with the problems inherent with this loss.

There are generally four different selves we portray in our lives. They are the community self, the worker self, the home self, and the private self. For each of these we have a different set of behaviors, clothing, activities, and language.

- Our community self is generally our most polite and potentially artificial self. It is developed throughout our life and generally guided by parents, teachers, and social norms. When we are in this role we tend to wait in line, hold doors open for others, and maybe most importantly, bite our tongues when we have a thought that isn't socially acceptable to share.

- Our worker self is often similar to our community self; however, it tends to be more focused as well as filtered. Our behavior related to this self centers more around the interactions with, and expectations of, supervisors, colleagues, and possibly customers.

- Our home self is a more relaxed version that we share with those we are most comfortable with; this could possibly include family members and close friends. This self tends to be less filtered and we may say things that our community self or worker self would find too risqué. We do this because we are with people who know us best and accept our words and actions without being offended or turned off.

- Our private self is our most honest and comfortable self. We typically only use this self when we are truly alone and therefore no one can judge us. This self may walk around the house in little to no clothing, drink straight from the bottle, or say anything that comes to mind.

How do we determine which self to use? We interpret the environment using our five senses and memories of similar experiences and what was expected. We engage our pre-frontal cortex which regulates impulse control, allows us to make decisions, and be logical, reasonable, and rational. In addition, the prefrontal cortex allows us to be aware of ourselves but also to see the perspective of others. Our memories and thinking skills allow us to determine the presence of others, the identity of these people, the meaning of their non-verbal behaviors, the meaning of their words, and their tone of voice. These abilities also help us identify which activities could or should be done here, the types of things we have done here before, and our emotional responses to these activities. Once we figure all of this out, we select our persona and put it on. We then function as that self until there are cues and information to indicate that we should change which self we are using.

So, what goes wrong with this system when dementia strikes?

To understand how the two issues are related, it is important to review some of the key features of most dementias. Difficulty with impulse control, difficulty with immediate memory and recall, problems with language interpretation and abstract comprehension, difficulty with higher order problem solving skills, and impairment of mental flexibility are all hallmarks of early dementia.

- The person can't always restrain the desire to say or do what they would like rather than what is socially expected of them.
- The person does not get the message being sent in the words and phrases being used due to inaccurate or inadequate connections between semantic memories and the current event.
- The person can no longer reason through a complex social situation or unfamiliar environment and so makes errors in behavior based on partial understanding or faulty cause and effect reasoning.
- The person loses the ability to look at the situation from multiple viewpoints as well as the ability to take familiar information and reorganize it and categorize it in a new or unusual way.

The result is that the person is forced to use only the more routine and familiar responses regardless of the situation due to an inability to be flexible.

As the disease progresses these deficits in function become more and more pronounced. Additionally, long-term memories become less available and accurate. The ability to distinguish actual historic events from what might have been wished for or dreamed of is greatly diminished and the person begins to confabulate. Confabulation is the brain's way of filling in the gaps for missing pieces to make sense of what is happening. It isn't lying – the person thinks they are telling the truth. Their brain is doing the best it can to figure out what is happening, even when this differs from *your reality*.

The person is also experiencing impairments in visual perception and auditory comprehension that affect everything they see and hear. The more basic cognitive functions also begin to deteriorate. Attention and concentration are impacted. This makes it difficult for the person to remain focused, resulting in distractibility or inattentiveness to the most important facets of the environment or situation.

This also makes it problematic to change the focus of attention or activity, resulting in repetitive words and phrases or behaviors and actions, or even lack of initiation. These changes eventually destroy the ability to recognize people, places, objects, familiar routines, and consequently what should be done where, when, and with whom. It makes it nearly impossible to know which **self** to use at any given time.

One of the first behaviors that causes concern is when a person displays inappropriate behavior in public places. They may be at a luncheon and talk about how boring the speaker is, even though the speaker is within earshot. They may describe their caregiver as "that fat girl, over there." They might tell their spouse of 40 years, "I wish you would go home because I want to watch this show and you are bothering me." In other words, they no longer can recall and adhere to the rules of politeness. As the disease progresses, it becomes more and more difficult for them to figure out which self to use and it also becomes more difficult to sustain a public or work self for any length of time due to worsening impulse control and decreasing interpretative skills.

If I can't recognize you as my daughter, I will not take on my family self. If I have been using my private self, I may continue to use it in a very public situation. In this case, I may reach across the table to take your dessert because I don't see mine or because I ate mine and would like some more. It is at this stage we often hear family members and caregivers say that their loved one would never have done something like this. We hear that this person was always very soft-spoken and gentle and never yelled, swore, or got angry at anyone, no matter what. In these cases, it is probable that the person had these thoughts and was able to control them or, when in the privacy of his or her own space, did have these very reactions, BUT that he or she never let it show in any other situation.

With the onset of the disease, however, the person is no longer able to contain those words, thoughts, feelings, or reactions and they are now being used in family, work, and public situations.

In other situations, a typically social and engaged person may begin to refuse invitations, sit silently at gatherings, ask to leave soon after arriving, or discontinue relationships and activities that have been a major part of their life and purpose in living.

On the other hand, the person who had the greatest consistency between his or her private self and family, work, and public selves will tend to have the least change in behavior. In these situations, we typically hear family members and caregivers say, "She has always been that way!" or "That's just mama, she's like that!"

Here are some tips for care partners and family members to improve the quality of life for the Person Living with Dementia (PLwD):

- Make cues stronger and more consistent. If going out for lunch, put on dress up clothes and go to a quiet place. If bathing, have a warm comfortable space, use other familiar and habitual routines to lead up to the event, keep your tone and approach friendly and intimate.

- Reduce the number and frequency of role change demands. Use *your*-**self** to foster the use of *their*-**self**.

- Provide opportunities for using these *selves*.

- Use valued cues to elicit the *self* most desired in the situation. When the public, work, or family self becomes unusable, stop setting up situations that require one of them as that can result in frustration when the person is not able to perform. ALWAYS respect the person and appreciate the unique self you are seeing and experiencing.

Tips for family members and care partners to understand what is happening:

- Knowledge is the key to stress reduction. Begin to recognize and appreciate the different selves you have and use almost effortlessly. Learn about the changes that happen when someone develops dementia and how this might impact expectations, interactions, interests, relationships, and outcomes.

- Imagine the value and importance of various cues, props, and environmental supports in helping or hindering various self-expressions when internal systems are failing. Learning to match what care partners would like to see, with cues that foster those performances are essential.

- Talk openly about the need to reduce the demand for

using selves the person may no longer be able to master as the disease progresses.

Here's an exercise to build awareness of your own selves:

Consider the self you share or reveal to others. What personal information do you share:

- with someone you have never met before
- with a co-worker or colleague
- with a spouse, close friend, or significant other

Does that information change if you know it will be kept private or shared with a group?

What about the words you write in a letter or personal journal? Would they be different if you knew someone else would be reading it?

Think about how your responses vary and your emotions change as the situations differ.

What does this mean for the person living with dementia and those living around them?

What if YOU were to develop dementia? Think about the value of the old saying "…to thine own self be true…thou canst not then be false to any man." (*Hamlet,* spoken by Polonius, written by William Shakespeare)

In other words, practice being yourself now! Have you identified potential partners to share important aspects of your private self in some fashion, so that if you were not able to speak for yourself, you would have an ally? Planning for a *what if* scenario can make all the difference if undesired brain changes or life changes were to happen.

CHAPTER 4

What's Under the Hood?
The Primitive Brain Takes on
the Thinking Brain

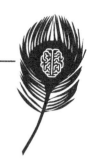

Humans are equipped with two major systems in their brains. They are the **primitive** brain and the **thinking** or **cortical** brain. Both are vital for humans, and yet each is unique. The two systems are developed separately and linked by wiring. It is the integration and balance of the two that allows us to function as we do in our roles and lives. A healthy balance results in a well-running human being that responds well to changing situations and can live well. The primitive brain handles the basics and emergencies. The thinking brain copes with the complexity of decision making, interpreting social and environmental messages, language, signals, and investigating possible solutions and new situations.

The first brain system to develop and come online is the **primitive brain**. It is developed in utero and has some basic functions that are active at birth. It continues to develop during the early years of life, reaching full function somewhere in the person's twenties. The primary functions of the primitive brain are designed to help with survival. This system is deep in the brain and governs the core functions of the human body through hard wiring into the parts of the brain that control respiration, blood pressure, blood sugar, heart rate, temperature control, wake/sleep cycles, recognition and reaction to pain, digestion, elimination, hormonal control, and internal sensations such as hunger, thirst, discomfort, and emotional distress.

This part of the brain is also referred to as the **limbic system** or the **reticular activating system**. Some of the structures that are involved in the primitive brain are:

- medulla oblongata (brain stem)
- amygdala (threat perceiver and pleasure seeker)
- thalamus and hypothalamus (central station for all entering and exiting nerve fibers that go to/from the spinal cord)
- basal ganglia
- hippocampus (left and right)

The overall purpose of this part of the brain is to keep the person ALIVE. To keep the person's core rhythmic functions going whether awake, asleep, or unconscious is one life sustaining function. A second function is the ability to react quickly in dangerous situations and to find moments of pleasure and satisfaction while living. To live well, the primitive brain must function well and consistently. The system never totally shuts down, it is always on, operating more like a dimmer switch than an on/off light switch.

The thinking brain develops as a baby transitions into a child, then into a teenager, and then becomes a young adult. As the system matures, the person continues to experience the world and build more and more elaborate connections between and among pieces of the puzzle of incoming data. This part of the brain is called the **cortex**. It has multiple lobes or areas of function. Each is primarily devoted to selective data intake, processing, and output. Each section, or lobe, is also wired into other sections and lobes and is wired into the primitive system in some ways.

- The **occipital lobes**, located at the back of the brain, handle visual input and processing. They are hard wired with your eyes through the optic nerves. They are also wired into the sensation-movement cortex, the balance coordination area (cerebellum), the language association area, and the temporal lobes for sound location.

- The **temporal lobes**, located over your ears, handle and process auditory incoming data, and are connected to the auditory nerve coming from your inner ear.

This section also forms and handles the emotional memories and interpretation of emotional data. Additionally, it helps you recognize people by their facial features, attach a name, and recall your relationship and feelings about them.

- The **frontal and parietal lobes** combine to support the connections between your body and your brain for sensation in and movement out. They are primarily wired through the spinal cord with connections through the primitive brain. There is a lot of cross-over wiring in this area called the **corpus callosum** to allow one side of the brain and body to work with and process alongside the other. Additionally, there are also strong linkages to the cerebellum, the vision center, and part of the nerve that comes from your inner ear called the vestibular nerve.

There are actually four distinct areas, and other associated areas, for primary sensation and movement. The last area of the thinking brain to develop and come online is referred to as the pre-frontal cortex.

- The **pre-frontal cortex** handles the most complex tasks in the thinking brain. It is responsible for taking all of the incoming data and working with it to process all this information and explore options, reach a reasonable conclusion, decide on a course of action, and then act, while evaluating the outcome, weighing in on how well it went, personal performance, possible alternatives, and evaluating how it might have impacted the larger environment and those around the person.

So how does all of this work in real life? Well, it all depends. The primitive brain is always in gear since it has to run things. At low levels, whether we are awake or asleep, it is the primary operator, if we believe we are in a low threat and satisfying situation. When we are in this friendly, familiar, functional, and forgiving place, our primitive brain is able to be alert and aware. It can focus more on meeting the basic requirements for living and in satisfying routine maintenance needs such as healing, growing, digesting, eliminating, recalling, and playing with information about pleasurable or unpleasant experiencing during REM sleep, and practicing our interaction with others who are within the *family/intimate* group.

If we are in less familiar, less comfortable, less friendly, or less functional situations, the primitive brain is ramped up a bit. It is now more vigilant of possible threats to safety and well-being and is more actively seeking to get *wants* met and making sure it is getting what it is lacking in the moment. In this state, the primitive brain is working with the **thinking brain** to take in, process, and respond to data. This is when humans will be exploring new environments, seeking out that which they are interested in, figuring things out, getting satisfaction from experiencing sensations, events, activities, and interactions that use abilities in creative, new, interesting, or entertaining ways. Learning and emotions are engaged and although the person may feel challenged, there is a sense of achievement or fulfillment in the experience.

If we believe we are in an unsafe or dangerous situation, the primitive brain takes over! It becomes the boss of the brain and body! It commands and dominates the entire system until safety is found or the system can no longer function. In this state, the primitive brain is using the core engine and arousal system to keep the human being alive. The person becomes hyper-vigilant, hyper-alert, and is in fright, flight, or fight mode. The primitive system overrides and limits the abilities of the **thinking brain** in order to get the person to safety, to drive the person to preserve the life of another, and/or to save that which the person believes is vital to their survival. It is fascinating, however, that a more mature brain can OPT OUT if it is able to determine that the situation is actually only **risky, not dangerous**. This happens as a result of experience, skill, or rehearsal. Simulations and practice of potentially dangerous interactions, situations, and experiences can and do build connections between the primitive and thinking brain that promote more thoughtful and skillful responses rather than automatic reactions. Through the teens and twenties, the brain is very busy creating this new wiring system. It is a critical time for developing this ability to be thoughtful and responsive rather than just reactive. It is essential that the brain be challenged, but not overwhelmed. It is also a high-risk time for shortcuts to pleasure.

This can lead to a lifelong struggle to differentiate between what is liked and wanted versus what is needed to create joy and fulfillment. Think about a New Year's resolution to become more physically fit. You need to set small goals and be consistent. It takes time, support, encouragement, and yet some opportunities for errors, mistakes, and failure, to create the wiring and firing within the system to optimize the brain into an effective management system.

So, in many forms of dementia, there is damage **early** in the condition to the learning and memory part of the hippocampus, the primitive brain, and the sensory intake and processing portions of the thinking brain. These changes can cause the primitive brain to sense threat where there is none, and yet miss the real dangers that do exist. It can make it difficult for the person to be aware that changes are coming from within themselves, rather than the external world, since their core system is not fully functioning and is actually *lying* to them. These changes can also cause the primitive system to switch to DANGER or NEED mode when neither situation is real.

By the **mid-stages** of dementia, the failure of both systems creates a new challenge for all involved. The person may or may not remember events from moment to moment and they may attach old experiences and events to new ones in unexpected and potentially dangerous or distressing ways. The inability of the brain to determine what is safe and unsafe, or items and experiences that are liked versus needed, can cause care partners to trigger their own primitive brain reactions if they are not able to override their systems and think it through.

By the **late-stages** of the condition, the primitive brain is struggling to hold it together. It is not able to cope with all the internal destruction and missing wiring, and control over the body's functions are falling apart. Survival is more and more difficult. Ultimately, the primitive brain is simply not able to manage all of the systems and the person is not able to stay alive. The body's core functions are failing. Yet, the system still has ways in which to protect the human: going into a sleep state, stopping the intake of food and drink, seeking out a place of comfort and familiarity. When this happens, the brain releases its own chemical cocktail that can calm and satisfy. In these moments that person may be alert and aware for brief periods and may be able to use the remaining thinking brain for short moments.

Appreciating the importance of the **primitive** and the **thinking brain** is vitally important to care partners. By using our mature and well-wired brain, we can support the person in ways that make sense and create the *just right* match to what they are and are not able to understand or do. When it works for everyone involved, it makes life worth living. **The most important questions to ask yourself:**

- Do I see opportunities, or do I feel threatened?
- Can I learn the skills needed to feel competent and able, or am I overwhelmed and frustrated?
- Can I let go of how things used to be to appreciate what is possible in this moment?

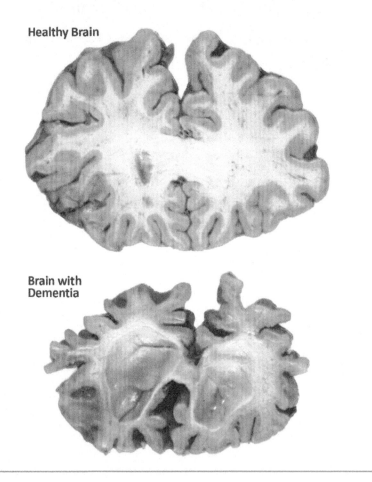

Pre-Frontal Cortex
Executive Control Center

- Impulse Control
- Being Logical
- Making Choices
- Self-Awareness

- Start – Sequence – Complete – Move On
- Seeing Another Point of View

Healthy Brain

Brain with Dementia

Graphic 6

The images are used with permission from *Alzheimer's: The Broken Brain,* Education and Training Program 1999, University of Alabama, Tuscaloosa

This photo shows the very front of the brain as though we had sliced off the front section and were standing in the person's shoes and looking at the slice from the inside out. We are seeing the wiring and storage sections that make up the frontal and pre-frontal cortex. The **top image is a healthy brain** with complete wiring (white matter) and massive amounts of storage capacity (gray matter). We can see just a hint of a ventricle in the left white matter. The **lower picture shows the ultimate result of Alzheimers**. The wiring is nearly gone. The ventricles are huge, storage capacity is limited, and getting information in and out is challenging and erratic. The desire to be respected and listened to is not necessarily affected, but the ability to use executive control systems is nearly impossible.

These images can be incredibly helpful in our understanding of why there are so many changes in ability. **For all that is lost, there are many pieces and parts that are still present, but not available or functional without support.**

One important thing to always recall, however, is that although two-thirds of the brain tissue may be missing, **there is still one-third present**. So, always keep in mind that "I am still here, until my brain can no longer get my body to do all that must be done to survive."

CHAPTER 5

Amygdalae and Brain Change—
Fright, Flight, or Fight

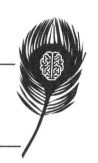

Our primitive brain contains two amygdalae. These structures are hardwired into our system to help us **survive**! Our
amygdalae have multiple roles. The primary one is that of a
threat perceiver, while another role is that of helping to get
needs met, and finally there is the role of pleasure seeker. The
roles combine to keep us alive, keep us out of danger, help us
find what we need to survive, and drive us toward moments
of pleasure, satisfaction, and joy.

The amygdalae (plural of amygdala) serve as sentries to **alert
us** of incoming dangers or risky situations, as well as guide us
in ways we get our **needs** met and **pleasures** found and ful-
filled. When sensing **danger**, these structures immediately
take control over the inner engine system and send a **rush** of
chemicals (adrenaline and cortisol) throughout the body to
provide what is helpful in emergency situations where quick
reactions might help us survive. We will have incredible

strength, greater speed, intense focus, and lack of pain awareness, in addition to heightened alertness, arousal, blood pressure, blood sugar, heart rate, and reaction speed. All of this is designed for escape or to overwhelm or eliminate that which threatens when there is a clear and present danger. It helps when death or severe injury is imminent.

The system also triggers when we have needs to be met. The goal is to grab nourishment and hydration when food and drink are available, to seek a safe place to eat, and to rest and recover. The amygdalae are the structures that crave the regular release of chemicals that give pleasure, such as endorphins, serotonin, dopamine, and oxytocin. The amygdalae also crave chemicals that give excitement, such as adrenaline.

The tricky part is that, once the amygdalae find *something* that gives immediate pleasure or relief, that *something* can become a needed and much sought-after item, although it is actually problematic in the bigger picture. Thus, they are a key player in addictive behaviors such as alcohol or drug consumption, gambling, overeating, sexual activity, speeding, extreme sports, or over-exercising. The rush of excitement can become so sought after that safety is abandoned.

Meeting Physical Needs to Avoid Distress

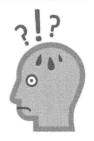

Intake:
- Hunger or Thirst
- Hydration—Nourishment
- Medications

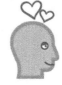

Comfort:
- Liking or not liking sensations, surfaces, social situations, or settings

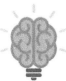

Energy:
- Wake-Sleep
- Tired
- Revved Up
- Focus Inward—Outward

Pain Free:
- Body pain *(joints, soft tissue, skin, more)*
- Emotional pain
- Spiritual pain

Elimination:
- Getting rid of excess or waste products *(urine, feces, sweat, saliva, mucus, hair)*

Don't forget to look in the mirror, sometimes we are the one with an unmet need!

Graphic 7

One final strength of the amygdalae is that they use their strong connection to the hippocampal areas to **remember** what feels good and to avoid that which was uncomfortable, risky, or potentially dangerous. They guide us back to places and situations where we found pleasure before, and they push the hippocampi (hippocampi is the plural of hippocampus) to increase the frequency of pleasure moments and slow down possible painful episodes. These small structures, in fact, play a *huge* role in how we live each and every day. The function and malfunction of the amygdalae system will create challenges in care support and environmental support when someone is living with dementia. When we combine the abilities of these two structures with the malfunctioning hippocampi, crises *seem* to be happening when and where they are not, and yet major problems occur when and where someone sees none! In almost all dementias, there are changes in the hippocampal areas of learning and remembering the details of new things, wayfinding from place to place and back, and keeping up with the passage of time.

Damage to the hippocampi tricks the amygdalae into acting quickly, and often with erroneous information, even early in the condition:

- The touch on your shoulder was not an attack, just your spouse trying to get your attention while you are online.

- It has actually been two days, not two hours, since you took a shower.

- You are driving, and missed the first turn in a series of four, so now you are panicking and angry because nothing is where it should be, and you can't get your brain to reason it out.

- Perhaps an older habit of seeking out alcohol to deal with discomfort or pain may return with a vengeance, and when combined with limited ability to keep up with how much you have consumed, results in brain-damaging binge drinking, without your conscious desire to do so.

Later in the condition, the primitive amygdalae may well cause you to:

- Seek only glucose-rich (sugary) food sources because they give you a quick rush of energy and pleasure.

- Become totally intolerant of background noises in a common space or group gathering, as they can't be sorted out from foreground sounds and are frightening or overwhelming.

- View friendly efforts to help you change soiled or wet clothing as an attack or invasion, resulting in an all-out battle for existence.

One of the ways we describe the amygdalae is similar to a traffic light:

- Green – The threat perceiver is experiencing no threat at all. Any discomfort is being dealt with and needs are being met. The pre-frontal cortex is an active participant and the pleasure seeker is finding something that is liked.

- Yellow – The threat perceiver is on alert and sensing the potential need to fire up due to a strong possibility that there could be a threat to well-being. The pathway into the pre-frontal cortex is starting to shut down and the amygdalae is taking over control and limiting pathways to and from other cortical structures as well (language skills, expanded visual field, or more complex object recognition). If the pleasure seeker is not getting what it wants, there is a greater push to immediate gratification.

- Red – The threat perceiver is on high alert and ready to act. The amygdala has shut down connections to cortical intake and output functions. The pleasure seeker moves into a need state and there is an immediacy to it.

Scale of Emotional Distress

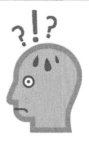

Typical Emotional Reactions to Stressors	Low *Amygdala Active* Alert	Medium *Amygdala Stressed* At Risk	High *Amygdala in Control* Endangered
Anger	Irritated Bothered	Angry Frustrated	Furious Enraged
Sadness	Dissatisfied Blue	Sad Unhappy	Devastated Hopeless
Loneliness or Feeling Forced	Missing *It*/ Not Getting *It* Missing Freedom/ Control	Lonely/ Disconnected Confined/ Restricted	Abandoned/ Isolated Imprisoned
Fearfulness	Nervous Anxious	Scared Worried	Terrified Panicked
Disappointment or Lack of Engagement	Disengaged Antsy	Bored Roaming	Useless/Purposeless Frantic

Graphic 8

The scales of distress (and excitement) are important to understand. Humans seek to be comfortable, pain free, and to avoid threats and danger, although they do need to find moments of joy and get their needs met to be satisfied!

In all cases, what is vitally important is that we appreciate the **power** of these structures in human beings. Our thinking and cognitively guided brains are not able to control these guys once they get in the **red zone**. When we are alert and aware, however, we can guide ourselves and the people we are trying to support through the use of distress-reducing techniques and likes/wants/needs-meeting strategies that keep each of us from approaching that **danger zone** of unmet needs. But it takes attention and skill. It requires us to take care of our brains and our bodies if we are going to be successful in the long run of supporting someone living with dementia from the beginning of the condition until the end of the journey. We will *need* to learn new ways of responding and notice when changes are making life distressing or pulling up old and risky coping strategies. We will actually require external monitors for our status, since we are in the middle of the situation and may be amygdalae-driven as well.

Here's another way to view the emotional scale of unmet needs:

Emotional States Affect All Brains

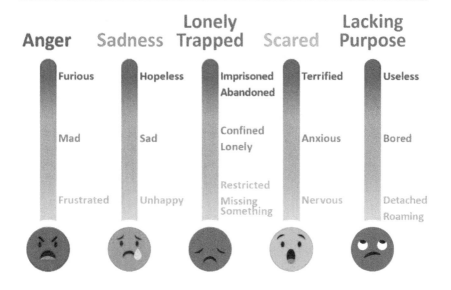

	Anger	Sadness	Lonely Trapped	Scared	Lacking Purpose
	Furious	Hopeless	Imprisoned Abandoned	Terrified	Useless
	Mad	Sad	Confined Lonely	Anxious	Bored
	Frustrated	Unhappy	Restricted Missing Something	Nervous	Detached Roaming

⬆ **Higher emotions =**
Primitive Reactions =
Fright, Flight, Fight, Hide, Seek

⬇ **Lower emotions =**
Responsive Brain =
More Thinking and Empathy

Graphic 9

Another piece of this amygdalae puzzle is that when the human brain changes *so much* that it no longer recognizes the need for sustenance for survival, the only reason the person continues to take a bite or take a drink is our relationship with them. We are frequently allowing *our* amygdalae to drive our interactions and demands on the *other* person. With a healthy brain, I would be starving if I didn't eat. I would be dying of thirst if I didn't drink something. The person living with dementia is not in the same state as we are. They aren't dying *because they aren't eating or drinking*. They aren't eating or drinking **because they are dying**. It is time for them to leave us. But, if we keep demanding that for our comfort they take in more, then they are only staying here for us. I believe we have the responsibility of asking ourselves and asking that person: "What have they **not** done that they **need to do** before they go?" Be truly curious about the possible answers, and attempt to solve the puzzle, if possible. And then, be prepared to allow the person to go or stay based on what you discover and can do.

Our amygdale are incredibly powerful parts of our brain that will stay with us until the end. They are designed to keep us alive, safe, and happy. Even with healthy thinking brains, they can get the best of us, but we need to learn to regain control and return to our thinking brain. We also will need to understand that when a person is living with dementia, the neocortex is one of the first pieces to go, which leaves the amygdalae in charge once more. When supporting someone living with dementia, we will need to do our best to keep both our amygdalae and our loved one's under control.

CHAPTER 6

Do You Hear What I Say? A Conversation Between Teepa and Tom

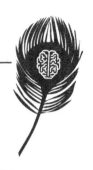

When someone is living with dementia, it is vital to appreciate the changes it makes in the person's ability to take in auditory data and make sense of it in a timely and effective fashion. Over the past few years, we have learned a great deal to heighten our appreciation of what is happening that changes the brain's ability to comprehend messages. This includes messages that are being received through hearing versus reading, in a crowded space versus a one-on-one situation, or even a familiar voice versus one that is unfamiliar. Other hindrances to comprehension include an unfamiliar accent or rhythm of speech, the switching of subjects, or when emotion is embedded in the content rather than just information or words. Speed, inflection, rhythm, and association with other sensory cues can totally modify how the meaning of the content is taken in and processed.

One critical element that is often missed when trying to share information with, or get information from, a Person Living with Dementia is the value of *changing our delivery process*. When we carry on traditional conversations we usually engage in a back and forth volley of information. As you can see in the example provided below.

In the first exchange, Teepa and Tom both have intact abilities in all areas of communication. Teepa is standing in the kitchen at the refrigerator and Tom is in the living room at his computer.

Teepa: *What do you want for dinner?*

Tom: *I'm not all that hungry. What do you have in the fridge that wouldn't be too much trouble and is lighter?*

Teepa: *It looks like I could do something with eggs or I could make a soup from left over vegetables and some canned beans I have.*

Tom: *How about an omelet with some of the veggies?*

Teepa: *Okay. Are you going to glass class after that? What time are you going to leave?*

Tom: *I need to pick up Jason and get pliers, so about 6:30 or so.*

Notice how one comment leads to the next and how the person getting the message internalizes it and then processes it and only then sends back a related but complex message of their own, moving the conversation and agenda forward for both of them.

In this second exchange, Tom has signs of language change that are consistent with Alzheimers in the early to mid-stages of the condition. Teepa is standing in the kitchen at the refrigerator and Tom is in the living room at his computer.

Teepa: *What do you want for dinner?*

Tom: *What?*

Teepa: *(louder) What do you want to eat tonight?*

Tom: *I'm going out tonight.*

Teepa: *I know that. I wanted to know what you wanted to eat for dinner.*

Tom: *I have **gas** class tonight. I've got to take something with me. Do you remember what it is?*

Teepa: *I'm not talking about that right now. I'll tell you later. Right now I want to know what you want for dinner!*

Tom: *Well, it sure **sounds** like you are talking to me right now! I don't remember what it is I'm supposed to take to class, but it is something that I need. I better call the guy who is going with me and see if we are going to get dinner on the way there.*

Teepa: *(comes to the living room doorway and puts her hands on her hips and raises her voice, sounding both frustrated and a little angry.) What are you talking about?! You are going to eat here, before you go to* **GLASS** *class. Jason is going with you and you have to get your* **PLIERS** *out of the workshop before you go. Now for the last time, what do you want to* **EAT** *for dinner?*

Tom: *Nothing! I'm not hungry. Why are you yelling at me?!*

When one person gets dementia, it is important to realize that the three language skills that are essential for processing and sharing verbal messages will need to be isolated and supported as unique and special skills. The three core skills are:

- Vocabulary (the words – the meaning of the content)
- Comprehension (receptive language – the ability to GET the message)
- Speech production (expressive language – the ability to GIVE the message)

It is also important to understand that various dementias can affect these processes in very different ways. Alzheimers disease is not the same as vascular dementia, which is also not the same as what is experienced with primary progressive aphasia, or frontotemporal dementia. Picking up on retained abilities and missing pieces can make all the difference in the world when trying to interact and support someone who is having trouble in one or more area.

It is vital to appreciate that there are often preserved or retained abilities that can support or help when trying to get a message across or obtain desired information from someone. These skills are related to rhythm skills and include:

- Social chit-chat – the back and forth that can mask loss of comprehension, but covers in short simple conversations
- Modulation of speech – this includes awareness of the changes in pitch or tone indicating a question or statement, as well as the ability to sustain rhythm or hear rhythm that sounds familiar
- Rhythmic speech such as music, poetry, prayer, counting, and even spelling

Additionally, changes in frequency, intensity, or volume can indicate shifts in emotional state or discomfort.

Learning to provide combination cues that use visual, verbal, and tactile data can enhance messages and promote better comprehension. Slowing down the exchanges and using reflective speech as well as pauses and simplified options can result in very different exchanges.

There are three important supportive phrases that can help when they are used in combination with pauses, inflections, visual cues, props, and partial reflective statements to confirm what was said or sought.

- Seek more non-specific information such as, "Tell me more" or "Tell me more about it."

- Seek demonstration or visual representation: "Could you show me how you would use it?" or "Could you show me what you would do with it?" or "Show me how you'd do it."

- Offer simplified options: either/or options that are exclusionary (all possible options fit into one grouping or the other) "Is it this or that?" or "Is it this or something else?"

Here is a repeat of the second conversation with these modifications:

Teepa leaves the kitchen to come to the living room doorway carrying a wooden spoon in her hand. She knocks on the door frame.

Teepa: *Hey Tom, sorry to interrupt.*

She pauses, making sure Tom is looking up at her before proceeding in the conversation.

Teepa: *I'm getting ready to fix dinner. Would you rather have soup or something else?*

Tom: *Soup or something else.*

Tom pauses and seems to be thinking.

Tom: *What's the something else?*

Teepa realizes Tom doesn't want soup, but is not sure what the other options are. She thinks through her other options.

Teepa: *So not soup, something else instead.... Hmmm, how about an omelet or a sandwich?*

Tom: *An omelet or a sandwich.... What's in the omelet?*

Teepa: *How about eggs and cheese and some veggies?*

Tom: *Eggs sound good and I love cheese, but what are veppies?*

Teepa: *So the eggs and cheese are good, but you aren't sure about the veppies? Let me show you what I've got and you can see what you think.*

Teepa goes to the fridge and gets out the leftover cooked broccoli and onions and brings them back to Tom.

Teepa: *Here are the things I have to put in with the eggs and the cheese for an omelet tonight.*

She pauses.

Tom: *Oh, those things are fine. I like them. I just didn't want those veppies you were talking about.*

Teepa: *Great. I'm going to get to work fixing this. Can you come and set the table?*

She gestures toward the kitchen and pauses, waiting for Tom to join her.

In this exchange, Teepa has mastered many skills, and uses them well. When Tom doesn't know what *veppies* are, she doesn't need to correct his miscomprehension of the word veggies. Instead, she gets what she has from the refrigerator to show Tom so he can make the choice. She has let go of the idea that specific vocabulary is needed for communication and that Tom can lob the conversational ball back over the net to her with each volley. She now uses more effective strategies to get the message in and to appreciate the message that is being sent.

Here is an image that depicts the changes in the left temporal lobe of the brain, the language center which controls vocabulary, comprehension, and speech production. The first picture is a healthy brain, while the second picture is of someone in late-stage dementia. What differences and similarities do you notice?

Left Temporal Lobe

Healthy Brain

Brain with Dementia

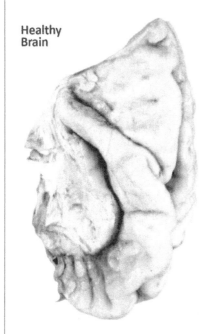
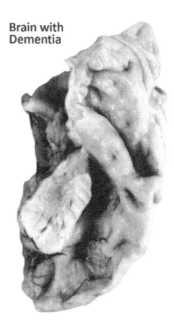

What do you notice has changed?
What has stayed the same?

Graphic 10

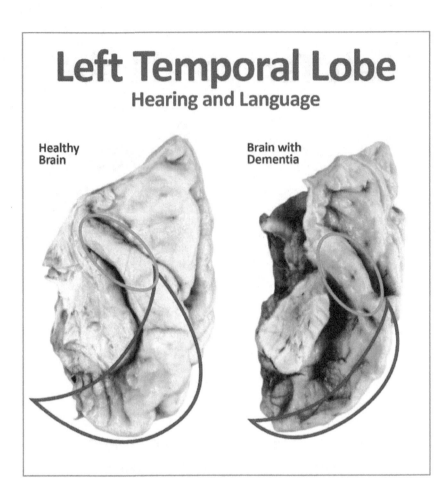

Graphic 11

The area outlined in blue is where the hearing function is located. It does not typically change with dementia. The biggest change in hearing is the ability to localize, to know where the sound is coming from, because that requires communication between the two sides of the brain where the wiring is damaged.

Look at the red shapes. There are drastic changes between the two images. This is where we keep our vocabulary, comprehension, and speech production functions.

When you are talking to someone and they say "What?" it is easy for us to assume they didn't hear us, so we speak more loudly. However, that won't be all that helpful if the problem is in the comprehension section rather than the hearing section. They may even ask you why you are yelling at them. What has changed is the person's ability to understand the words, know what those words mean, and create accurate words back to you.

There is one more piece to talk about, from Teepa and Tom's conversation which should not be overlooked. Teepa has one more BIG CHANGE to make; she needs to look inside and notice she has lost something. It's not there anymore and she is missing it. Sometimes more than others, but it is real and it is important. Her relationship with Tom is changing. She can't just throw out a conversational comment or idea and have him follow her lead. He is no longer taking a lead and giving her opportunities to follow. Teepa is having to actively think when she wants to communicate with Tom. Nothing is automatic anymore. Their companionship and partnership are not what they were.

So, two ideas:

1. Teepa and Tom may really benefit from creating opportunities and a schedule for episodes of fun and joy. Finding places in the day and in their life for music, poetry, song, dancing, playing instruments, or engaging in non-language related companionship or visually or physically oriented activities that both can share.

2. Teepa will want to develop some new or different opportunities to use her language skills and sustain her conversational talents and interests. Keeping herself satisfied with interactions and verbal exchanges will reduce the risk that she feels empty and depleted, so that her sharing with Tom is felt and seen as positive and fruitful, not repetitive or frustrating.

How will each of us learn to DO something new or differently that makes life a little better for those we care for and those who care for us?

CHAPTER 7

Changing Our Visual Awareness— What Do You See?

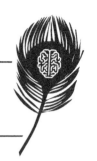

How we see things and how we perceive things are both very important in our daily lives. This applies to what we physically see with our eyes and our ability to see things from another person's perspective. Let's discuss both types of seeing: the physical components to seeing and how that changes with dementia as well as why it is so important to try and see things from another's perspective.

How do we get visual information into our brains? Visual data enters through our eyes, the light rays come through the cornea, cross the fluid in the eyeball and hit the retina, a photo-sensitive screen on the back of the eyeball. The rods and cones embedded in the layers of the back of the eyeball change the light rays into electro-chemical messages.

These messages are loaded into the optic nerve that comes out from a center point in the retina of each eye (your blind spot). The information is specifically sorted by quadrants for each eye. Then something extraordinary happens! Some fibers stay in their lane while others cross over at the optic chiasm.

This is what gives human beings the ability to have binocular (stereoscopic) vision as well as providing the opportunity for both depth perception and hand-eye coordination. In dementia, we now recognize the role of glial cell activity changes in the onset of dementia and its progression, as glial cells in the brain have a major role in maintaining the health and well-being of this ocular system. It makes sense, then, that changes in vision are typically going to be a part of the development of dementia.

The optic messages carried by these revised optic nerve bundles go through the thalamus, have connections to many other places and spaces, but ultimately most land within the occipital lobes of the cerebral cortex. From there they go to many other areas of the cortex, including the executive control center, the sensory-motor region, the vestibular and auditory processing areas, and much more. The fibers associated with vision are both widespread and powerful in human decision-making and behaviors.

There are some specific wiring patterns that exist and are important in daily function:

- The sight pathway wiring (seeing things)
- The vestibulo-oculo-reflex (balancing combined with vision – an example is the righting reflex – finding upright against gravity)
- The oculo-motor pathways (eye movement control)
- The dorsal stream (determining the *where* of objects, self, and movement)
- The ventral stream (determining the *what* that is seen and details of importance)

Although humans cannot begin to match eagles or other birds of prey for acuity, they do have fairly remarkable visual skills. They also have some unique wiring patterns that attach words to visual information, so that it can be shared among others when the item or thing being talked about is not actually present. I am going to give you a short laundry list of many of the visual abilities we use each day to make our world flow smoothly.

Driving a car uses a variety of these visual skills, so I have highlighted a few examples of how these specific skills are used.

- Visual Field - How much of the world can be taken in at any moment in time by the human visual system? There are four major areas – focused or targeted vision, central field vision, peripheral vision, and far peripheral vision (the outer rim of vision).

o Focused or Targeted vision is about an 8 degree circle from the middle of your vision, at a distance of about 18"- 36" from the eye.

o Central Field vision is the next 30 degrees to either side. It is about 36" wide at arm's length.

o Peripheral vision is another 30 degrees to either side and allows us to notice flashes of light, color, or movement, but not detail. For that we would have to adjust our eyes and head.

o Far Peripheral vision extends another 30-40 degrees. This is an area where we have awareness of movement and a range in which we are alerted of possible action, but a visual shift would have to happen for more information processing to occur.

Think about your visual field when you are driving and looking straight ahead. Even though your vision is directed to the central area, you are likely very aware of things that are happening to the sides.

- Accommodation – The ability to adjust near-to-far and far-to-near acuity. It typically happens very rapidly, within 220-250 milliseconds. The inability to see well at arm's length typically happens with increasing age.

Using the driving analogy again, think about how you shift your focus from the speedometer to a road sign coming up on the highway.

- Adaptation – The ability to adjust light to dark and dark to light conditions. This takes longer because it is mostly up to rods to do this work. It can take up to 20-30 minutes to fully adapt, so that color vision (cones) in limited light can still work.

While driving, your vision must adapt quickly when entering and exiting a tunnel that is not well lit.

- Depth Perception – The ability to use the integrated images from both eyes to judge depth, distance, figure-ground discrimination[3], 2-D versus 3-D images, and organize hands, feet, and body to prepare, respond, and adapt to changing features and surfaces.

A specific example of depth perception when driving is judging how quickly that oncoming car is approaching before you make a left turn?

---

[3] Figure-ground discrimination is the ability to discern where one object stops and another begins. Imagine looking into a messy kitchen drawer with utensils placed randomly. Figure-ground discrimination allows you to know that the pizza cutter is not part of the spatula which is not part of the salad tongs, despite all of them lying with one another.

- Organized Scanning – The ability to get the six muscles around each eye to collaborate and coordinate to move in a seeking pattern throughout a visual range, in order to find a pre-selected item or to locate an anomaly or unexpected element.
  - o Saccadic Eye Pursuit Movements – point-to-point or item-to-item looking is called saccadic (picking spots and ignoring things between the spots). This is used in reading, driving, walking, doing tasks, looking for something, and searching for things.
  - o Smooth Pursuit Eye Movements – smooth pursuit is used when tracking a moving object or following something with your eyes. It is rarely used if an item is not targeted.

Organized Scanning is used constantly while driving. For instance, as your focus shifts from the car ahead of you to your rearview mirror, to the road ahead.

- Visual Attention – The ability to attend to some visual information while seeming to ignore or not process other visual information that is available. It is subdivided into three categories:
  - o Sustained Visual Attention – ability to stay focused on a visual item or activity over time.
  - o Selective Visual Attention – ability to pick out

sought after or important visual data from background data.

   o   Divided Visual Attention – ability to switch back and forth from one visual focus to another or pay attention to multiple aspects or items in a visual field.

An example of visual attention while driving might be frequent shifting of attention from the pedestrian on the sidewalk, to the stop light, to the street sign.

- Color Vision – handled primarily by the cones that are concentrated in the more central part of vision. There are three cone shapes and each type handles one wavelength of light. Most are set for red, then green, and only a few pick up blue. People who are color blind have deficits in those cones. Loss of cones results in loss of ability to discriminate colors or accurately identify them.

- Object Recognition – This is a highly complex skill and still under intense investigation. It is the ability of humans to assign a purpose and value to an object both in and out of context. It is also involved in the person's ability to prepare to handle or use an object, based on past experience with that object or similar objects. If you have ever had a bicyclist swerve out into the roadway, your reaction as you approach a biker will be different than if you have never had this experience.

- Facial Recognition – This particularly specialized function in the human brain is where facial features are used to identify people. This regional system associates a name with a face. Problems with recognizing faces is called prosopagnosia. It turns out that infants are good at recognizing positive and negative emotions in facial expressions before they are able to recognize specific details for people identification. They also are more reactive to negative emotional features than positive emotions from an early age. The ability to assign a face to a familiar or unfamiliar category develops next. Finally, the child can identify specific persons of importance to them by about seven months of age.

- Visual-Motor Integration – This is the ability of the visual cortex to work with the sensorimotor cortex and the cerebellum to allow for smooth actions based on visual input and sensory motor feedback loops. Your passengers in the car will appreciate the smooth coordination of your transition from the gas pedal to the brake as you slow towards a traffic light!

- Visual-Vestibular Function – This refers to the wiring between the inner ear, the sensorimotor system, and the optic system to coordinate gaze, body movement, and equilibrium with gravity, constantly impacting what is done.

Since vision is such a vital part of sensory processing, changes brought on by dementia are incredibly impactful for a human being. Each of the functions listed above has the potential to be greatly affected by various forms of dementia. There are some areas spared with many dementias, while some dementias are particularly challenging for visual function.

Posterior Cortical Atrophy is a dementia that has a primary visual impact. It can and does rob a person of so many visual skills that function is often problematic even early on when symptoms first develop. What is more problematic, however, is that many of these cases are not diagnosed until the challenges are well advanced for the person and their support system.

People living with vascular dementia may have both a loss of one entire side of vision brought on by strokes, as well as problems with processing and visual-perception changes due to the cortical changes of their dementia.

Individuals with Lewy Body Dementia frequently experience visual activity that results in visual misperceptions or hallucinations as part of their condition, for instance, Capgras syndrome (the sense that a familiar person has been replaced by an imposter).

People with other forms of dementia may also experience visual hallucinations when in physiological or emotional distress.

Misunderstanding of hallucinations can cause acute health problems to be mismanaged or problematic medications to be used to treat a symptom of dementia, not a psychosis.

Because vision is so central to human actions, reactions, and behavior, it is especially important to notice the visual shifts that are taking place for the Person Living with Dementia and ensure that we use the abilities that remain in all that we do. There is so much that can and does go wrong with vision and visual abilities in the world of dementia, it is easy to miss how helpful the remaining visual abilities can be. Using visual cues and fewer words can help ensure that the message being delivered is the message being received.

We must also recognize the essential role our visual abilities will play in our interactions, our environmental considerations, and our responses to situations that arise.

In the world of dementia, being able to see things from another person's perspective is critical to successfully:

- Form relationships that work
- Initiate interactions that have value and meaning for both people
- Get important tasks completed with limited stress or distress
- Live lives that are fulfilling and provide moments of joy and pleasure

- Be part of a community that acknowledges the person, supports one another, celebrates victories, and most importantly, comforts in times of grief, loss, and sorrow

About two-thirds of all of our sensory processing is affected by visual data. There are about one million nerve fibers coming out of each eye. Eight of the twelve cranial nerves are somehow involved in visual processing. We use vision a great deal for most activities in which we engage or avoid. Control over our eyes is highly complicated and integrated, yet in some ways remarkably primitive. It is estimated that humans make decisions about liking or not liking another human being within seven seconds of visually regarding that person. Humans are well known for making snap decisions about meals or willingness to taste something, based on appearances.

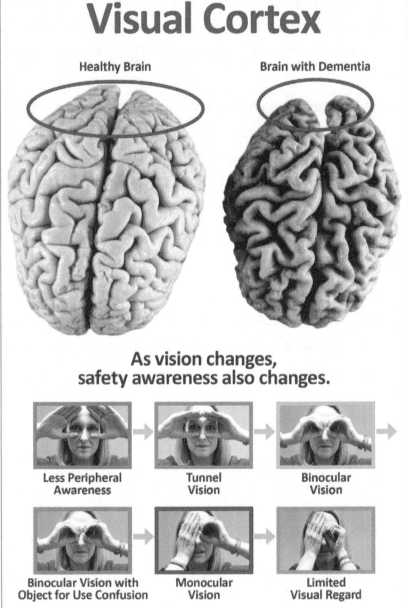

Visual Cortex

Healthy Brain **Brain with Dementia**

As vision changes, safety awareness also changes.

Less Peripheral Awareness → Tunnel Vision → Binocular Vision →

Binocular Vision with Object for Use Confusion → Monocular Vision → Limited Visual Regard

Graphic 12

Seeing things from the other person's point of view is not optional, but essential in dementia care, for the well-being of all involved. Making efforts to understand another perspective, trying out a task with limitations, consider how it might look if… are all possible ways in which we can improve our care support and setting for people living with various forms and degrees of dementia.

We will discuss the importance of visual cues as well as verbal and touch cues in the next chapter.

CHAPTER 8

Using Cues as a Care Partner— Cue Up a Successful Interaction

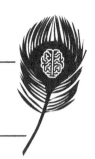

Throughout my career as an Occupational Therapist, I have conducted research and provided direct care to a wide variety of people, including those living with dementia. This has allowed me to learn how People Living with Dementia navigate their world when challenged by the effects of a changing brain. I would like to share with you some of my observations and some cues that can improve our work as care partners. Sensory systems (what a person sees, hears, feels, smells, and tastes) help human beings understand and interact with their world.

As we discussed in the previous chapter on vision, all people live in continuous cycles of taking in sensory data, processing, and then using that information. When someone has dementia, there is interference within the sensory processes. People living with dementia want to get along in the world, just like anyone else, and they are trying to figure out how to do that. When working with a Person Living with Dementia, you will encounter some challenging situations. What you might be experiencing is a breakdown in their sensory process. And while it might seem confusing and create frustration for you, this is likely a person's best attempt to understand and meet their own needs under the circumstances and with the abilities they are living with in that moment.

People need to stay engaged with the world around them, although their abilities to do so safely are being eroded. Eventually, due to the effects of dementia, those we are caring for will need our help to do this. The first and most important step is to observe. If you take the time to observe, you will often be able to discover the abilities a Person Living with Dementia possesses at any given moment. If we can understand more fully what someone *can* do, instead of focusing on what they *can't do anymore,* then we can choose to support and care for them in a way that will make sense. This begins with observations, rather than assumptions about what is happening.

Second, look for sensory cues. All human beings are giving us clues and information about their ability through their action or behavior with others and the environment. Take an inventory by honestly observing and respecting how the person living with dementia is relating to the world through their five senses. When you observe the person doing or not doing something, it will provide you with valuable information about them *and* their abilities. You might notice what that person is taking in from their environment, and any unmet needs they are attempting to satisfy.

5 Ways the Brain Takes in Information

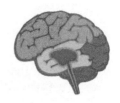

What You See:
- Visual data
- Taken in by the Eyes
- Processed by:
  Occipital Lobe

What You Hear:
- Taken in by the Ears
- Processed by:
  Temporal Lobe

What You Feel or Do:
- Sensory-Motor data
- Taken in and sent out through Skin, Muscle, and Joints
- Processed by:
  Frontal Lobe, Parietal Lobe

What You Smell:
- Olfactory data
- Taken in by the Nose
- Processed by:
  Frontal Lobe, Parietal Lobe, Limbic System *(deep in brain)*

What You Taste:
- Gustatory data
- Taken in by the Tongue
- Processed by:
  Frontal Lobe, Parietal Lobe

Graphic 13

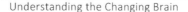

Visual cues –

Notice what a person is focused on. What can/do they see that might be different from what you are able to see? Visual cues are typically a human being's first method and favorite way to take in informational data. Over time, dementia causes many changes in the brain's occipital lobe, impacting a person's visual field, object recognition, figure-ground awareness, and depth perception. Due to these changes, a person literally may not know you are sitting next to them. They can't see you, even though you might be able to see them. If you have observed and are aware of this, then you can help by moving yourself into a person's visual field, at a personally comfortable distance, before attempting to communicate or provide support or care. Try starting from a distance of more than six feet away, in their visual field. Once eye contact is established, speak and move in closer, standing *slightly* to their side.

You can experiment with some of the changes that occur in the visual abilities of someone living with dementia.

To get a sense of what it might be like to have a limited ability to take in significant amounts of visual data at any moment in time, try limiting your peripheral visual fields. Put your hands around your eyes as though you are looking through binoculars. This approximates what you might be able to take in by the time you are in the mid-stages of dementia.

Try these two things by yourself:

1. With your binoculars on, look down at your shirt to determine if it is clean or dirty.
2. Put on your binoculars and carefully walk around your room, noticing what you see and don't see. Where is your vision focused as you walk around? What is your awareness of people and objects around you?

Try these with a partner to see which feels better:

- Now, have someone walk up to you from about twelve feet away and not stop until they are one arm's length (about three feet) from your face.
- Next, have them start from twelve feet away and stop moving at six feet away.

Which feels more comfortable to you with your limited peripheral vision?

- While you are watching them with your binoculars, have the person stand at one arm's length in front of you.
    - First, have them stand directly in front of you, so if either of you took a step forward, you would bump into each other.
    - Second, have them pivot outward on their left foot while stepping back on their right, so that

they end up standing to your right side, immediately next to your right shoulder. You may have to turn your head to see them. Now you are at a 90° angle, and if either of you took a step forward, you would simply cross in front of one another.

Thinking about your visual field with the binoculars on, which setup felt more comfortable?

How do these activities alter your awareness of peripheral vision and changes that can occur with dementia? What have you learned about the way you approach and stand near a person you are speaking with?

Think about the value of providing visual cues which give information and context about an activity, for example a jacket when it's time to go outside, or a comb when some grooming is needed. What visual cues could be used to offer choices to match your words, for instance, "Would you prefer the blue shirt or the red one?"

Auditory and Verbal cues –

If a Person Living with Dementia is speaking to you but their words are not readily available, misused, or misinterpreted, try to notice the rhythm, the intensity, the pattern, and the volume of what they are saying. Consider what they are saying or attempting to communicate with their actions, if not their words. Notice how they respond to you when you speak - or if they respond at all. A lack of response can also be a *cue* about ability in a particular moment. Did they hear you? Did they actually process what you said? Did you get a response that suggests they understood? What is happening in their body that might provide you with clues? In order to reduce your risk of making a mistaken assumption, try checking in. Do you have eye contact? Did they offer any words? If so, confirm you got them by saying their words back to them. Can you think of a gesture or object you could show the person to provide additional support for the message you were delivering or that indicates what you thought they answered? Matching your pace to their response time is important. You may need to give them 3-5 seconds or more to process your question and respond to you. Resist the urge to speak louder, repeat the question multiple times, or rephrase your question several times before they have an opportunity to respond. Consider the number of words they are offering you, and try to use similar patterns when communicating. Using facial expressions, gestures, demonstrations, or props are all helpful strategies to become more comfortable with, as comprehension and speaking abilities change.

Movement and Touch cues –

When you are observing a person, what are things that draw their interest, what is being avoided? What skill versus strength abilities are noted? Are skilled tasks such as doing buttons or zippers, taking the cap off the toothpaste, or using a utensil to eat becoming difficult? Could changes in these skilled abilities cause distress or possibly be a reason the person has stopped doing their personal care? Could changes in dexterity or sensation explain why objects or tasks are being avoided or poorly done? Is there an action or reaction to movement, touch, or stillness that is worth exploring or paying attention to? It helps to be aware that although people living with dementia exhibit curiosity, many lack a sense of safety awareness. Someone living with dementia, who is not aware of the changes they are experiencing may see our behavior and efforts to keep them safe as threatening or unnecessary. Not noticing and addressing safety concerns that occur with changing abilities represents one error, yet impulsive attempts to enforce limits without thoughtful observation and use of skills can turn a risky situation into a dangerous one in only a few seconds. Yelling someone's name across the room will be ineffective, and grabbing something out of their hand, or pulling them away from a door can cause significant, if unintended, negative consequences.

There will be more information about improving the cues we give for care in the books that follow, which will provide a guide for successful interactions. It's important to understand and be aware that over time there will be a change in almost all experiences of sensation for a Person Living with Dementia. This means changes in visual abilities, auditory processing, and comprehension ability. Although the person will not typically have a change in the ability to hear a sound, the ability to sort out background sounds from foreground sounds, to locate the source of the sound, and to interpret the value of the sound will definitely be impacted. Regarding the complex and interwoven world of touch and movement, abilities and interpretations will definitely be altered. The ability to feel and manipulate an object will be diminished. Both internal and external pain, discomfort, and pleasure signals can be misunderstood or lost. These can include light moving touch, deep pressure, temperature, and sharp/dull awareness. There can also be changes in the ability to accurately identify smells and tastes as well as changes in a person's awareness of dangers associated with particular situations or items. Every sensory experience is changing for the Person Living with Dementia. This impacts behavior, the giving and receiving of communication, and therefore, relationships with others. If we truly understand this, and are willing to observe and stretch ourselves by looking at what's happening through the lens of curiosity, we can then further understand and choose to support and care for others in ways that make more sense. These changes in perspective will improve relationships and assist in setting realistic goals for care partner interactions. Most importantly, these changes give the Person Living with Dementia - who is doing the best they can with what they have - a greater sense of value, individual choice, and sense of control throughout their life, as they are living it.

CHAPTER 9

Understanding Way Finding— How Do I Get There From Here?

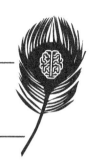

Humans, like many other creatures, have a built-in navigation system that allows them to find their way from one place to another AND return to the place from which they started. After much research and investigation, it turns out that this system is highly complex and is based deep in our brains in the hippocampal region, with wiring to many other locations. The hippocampus is well known as a high-risk area for loss of function when dementia hits. It is also responsible for learning new things and remembering them, as well as for the awareness of time (temporal orientation).

Different dementias affect the region in different ways, but many compromise our ability to use cues and traditional ways of knowing where we are and how to go to familiar places or return to the place where we started. The directions of turns, sequence of turns, and visual recognition from the reverse side of a landmark or location makes independent travel risky and difficult. The reality that it can hit you all at once that you don't know where you are, how you got there, or how to get home again can be both terrifying and overwhelming.

Wayfinding helps people living with dementia move independently from one spot to another. It refers to what people see, what they think about, and what they do when finding their way from one place to another[4].

How do we get from Point A to Point B and back again? By what means do we know how to find the bathroom? What about the extra toilet paper we bought last week? How do we get to our bank, the grocery store, a gas station, the dry cleaners, and back home?

Anyone familiar with *Still Alice*, either the book by Lisa Genova or the movie starring Julianne Moore, will probably recall the scene when Alice can't find her hotel and experiences a panic attack. Unfortunately for people living with many forms of dementia, this is an all-too-frequent and real experience. For those surrounding and supporting the person through these events, it can also be traumatic and overwhelming.

---

[4] Brawley, E. C. (1997). *Designing for Alzheimer's disease: Strategies for creating better care environments.* New York: Wiley.

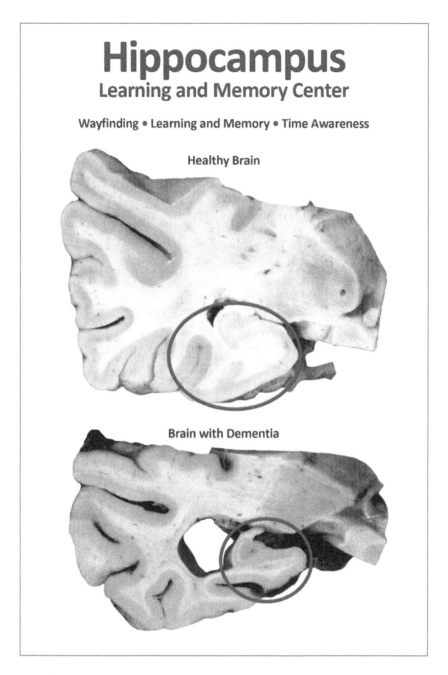

Hippocampus
Learning and Memory Center

Wayfinding • Learning and Memory • Time Awareness

Healthy Brain

Brain with Dementia

Graphic 14

When we try to use language and explanations to help, it doesn't. Increasing the number of times we say something or the volume at which we try to explain comes across as threatening and can make the situation worse. Instead of breaking the wall down, we are actually making it a more emotional event which places us on the opposing side rather than alongside the person in their fear, frustration, and distress. If we don't pause and reassess the situation, rather than trying to immediately help the person, our efforts can take the situation from one of risk to one that is out-and-out dangerous for the person, others, ourselves, and the environment. We can actually risk making new emotionally distressing memories. Memories get misfiled and are not filled in accurately with the right detail.

This results in challenges, as some memories of places and spaces that were once safe and familiar will now feel dangerous and should be avoided at all costs. These places may include bedrooms, bathrooms, dining tables, homes, and/or restaurants. The fear of getting lost can become so great that the person actually limits their efforts to leave their immediate environment, becoming less and less able to go out, be out for any length of time, and yet still not feel comfortable at home either. Hence the need to leave and try to find home without getting caught. Or perhaps the fear of letting anyone in and distrusting even the closest friends or family members.

As dementia continues to progress to mid-stage, it becomes

harder and harder for the person to use environmental cues to guide and direct movement from place to place, from location to location, or even from home to another familiar place and back with consistency. This phenomenon plays a major role in the potential for elopement and wandering that is documented in dementia. Between 60-70% of everyone living with dementia will at one time or another leave a location unexpectedly and become lost or missing. People Living with Dementia represent the second most common population to experience getting lost. Children are first on the list. This results in massive numbers of volunteer call outs for search and rescue, as well as enormous time and monetary costs to the public service providers, not to mention the emotional costs to all involved. Increasing the safety net and recognizing the need for advance thinking and planning is important for the possibility, or even probability, of the Person Living with Dementia becoming lost or leaving on an emotional mission and becoming disoriented in both place and time.

So, how can we provide support and help as the internal system of wayfinding becomes less and less reliable?

As the disease progresses, it changes the person's ability to know what to do, where to do it, when to do it, and when to transition to do something else, somewhere else. Because of this, it will become necessary to change either who is available to help or where the help is delivered. A new environment, or a change of people in the environment, can be stressful on all involved. However, avoiding a much-needed change can also heighten the risk of injury or incidents, isolation, or disengagement. In addition, it removes the opportunity for becoming comfortable in a different place or situation while there are still possibilities to get the *feel* for the new place and people, even if the details don't stick.

Here are some helpful suggestions for supporting a person's ability to get around by using some environmental strategies.

Effective wayfinding cues[5]:

- Landmarks – a particular tree or garden bed
- Interior and exterior decorating schemes
- Sculpture, paintings, or other decorative features
- Planned architectural features like personalized doorways
- Changes in color
- Changes in lighting levels
- Changes in floor surfaces

How can we help?

- Keep signs simple as people may no longer be able to understand complex language or writing
- Place signs at eye level for those using wheelchairs

---

[5] http://www.health.vic.gov.au/dementia/strategies/wayfinding.htm

- Use bright contrasting colors
- Personalize room entries to make them more relevant to individuals
- Create a regular schedule so daily life experiences are in the same place at the same time of day
- Create purpose specific rooms so people know what to expect when they enter them
- Make key places such as dining rooms, bathrooms, and living rooms easily seen

For an additional resource which compares the impact of dementia on wayfinding by GEMS State with intervention suggestions, please use this QR Code.

Scan this code with your smartphone's camera or visit **www.teepasnow.com/moreinfo** on your computer.

How we choose to help can make a major difference for all of us involved in the ability to adjust and adapt.

Finally, it is always important to know that at the end of a person's time on this earth and their residence within the temporary house we call their body, it is still important to provide that which feels like a safe haven. It is the assurance that when I can no longer function within my house, you can provide the friendship, familiarity, and forgiveness that allows me to know I can let go and move on. That you will miss me, still love me, and honor me. And most important, that in letting go, I am not giving up and neither are you. You are simply offering me the opportunity to find release and completion, acknowledging that our work is done, and all will be well for all of us.

CHAPTER 10

Wandering—Am I There Yet?

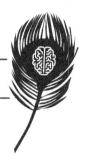

Wandering is defined as moving from place to place without a fixed plan; roaming, rambling. When dementia is involved, unsupervised wandering is dangerous and more common than you might think. **Six out of ten people with dementia will wander.** A person with Alzheimers or another form of dementia may not remember his or her name or address and can become disoriented even in familiar places.

Who is at risk of wandering?

Anyone who has memory problems and is able to walk is at risk for wandering. Even in the early stages of dementia, a person can become disoriented or confused for a period of time. It's important to plan ahead for this type of situation. Wandering and getting lost is common among people with dementia and can happen during any stage of the disease.

Be on the lookout for the following warning signs:

- Returns from a regular walk or drive later than usual
- Tries to fulfill former obligations, such as going to work
- Tries or wants to *go home*, even when at home
- Is restless, paces, or makes repetitive movements
- Has difficulty locating familiar places like the bathroom, bedroom, or dining room
- Asks the whereabouts of current or past friends and family
- Acts as if doing a hobby or chore, but nothing gets done (for example: moves around pots and dirt without actually planting anything)
- Appears lost in a new or changed environment

There are local and national organizations that provide programs and devices to assist in location monitoring for those who wander. There is an assortment of options to aid in safety and tracking – devices worn around the neck, smart watches/wristbands, even devices that fit inside a shoe – to name but a few. These devices can help people feel safe and connected. Some contain GPS locater signals to help find those that may wander.

As a care partner, now that you know the warning signs, how can you limit the risk of wandering? Here are some tips from the Alzheimer's Association website:

- Provide opportunities for exercise to reduce anxiety, agitation, and restlessness
- Ensure all basic needs are met (toileting, nutrition, thirst)
- Carry out daily activities such as folding laundry or preparing dinner, to provide daily structure
- Reassure the person if he or she feels lost, abandoned, or disoriented
- Avoid busy places that are confusing and can cause disorientation such as shopping malls
- Place deadbolts either high or low on exterior doors (only if you are home with the person living with dementia)
- Control access to car keys (a person living with dementia may not just wander by foot)
- Do not leave someone living with dementia unsupervised in new surroundings
- Consider sensitively telling local shopkeepers and neighbors whom you know and trust about the person's dementia and give them your contact details - they may be able to keep a look out

- If the person is in a day or activity program, respite residential care, or long-term care, tell the staff about their tendency to walk about. You can also ask about the home's policy on safe walking and care for residents who are prone to wander about

If the person does wander, consider these tips that increase the likelihood of a positive outcome:

- The care partner should consider carrying a card that says, "I'm a caregiver of someone living with dementia."
- Make sure the person carries some form of identification or the name and phone number of someone who can be contacted if they get lost. You could sew this into a jacket or a handbag so that it is not easily removed.
- If the person uses a mobile phone, ensure that the phone number of the primary care partner is stored and is easily accessible. If the mobile phone is switched on, it may be possible to trace the person if they are missing.

What Not to Do:

If you are leaving a person living with dementia alone in a home, apartment, or building while knowing that the person would not be able to safely exit the building in case of a fire or emergency, it is considered neglect. It is important to begin making alternate arrangements and seeking assistance or support to make sure, as a care provider you can do what you need to do, while the person receives the monitoring they need in your absence.

It is not a safe practice to rely on medications such as sleeping aids to keep the person from getting up at night. Doses heavy enough to stop someone from waking or walking can increase the likelihood of falls, cause incontinency, increase confusion, and cause memory problems. Additionally, some individuals are so unable to sleep or so driven to move about that the medications do not work consistently. There is a critical need to make sure there is a safety net of a secured setting to reduce the risk of fall related injuries or unobserved exiting or elopement.

CHAPTER 11

Repetition—I Might Have Told You This Already, But...

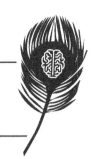

Here is what gets me curious...

Why do people repeat the same actions, words, or interactions over and over?

Why is it that some people seem to find comfort in the repetitions and others find them annoying or irritating?

What makes the difference?

What would be something different that works for both participants?

What can we do to alter interactions so that what happens is okay and we get something different to happen rather than staying stuck in a repeating loop?

How do we get it to take place?

What we know about human brains, their development, function, and failure, informs us a good bit about why people repeat things. Repetition typically happens when:

- I am trying to learn something new. It turns out I am creating a new synaptic pathway for future and continued use. Repeating something multiple times strengthens the firing sequence for neurons and makes it easier for me to follow the pathway without having to seek it out. It changes it from something that has to be thought about (pre-frontal) and processed as a separate element to a new automated pattern:
  - words = temporal= hippocampal
  - motions-sensations = parietal-frontal-hippocampal
  - visuals = occipital-hippocampal
- I have determined that this new data or process is important to my well-being, for some reason. This is something important to me! If it is important, then I will try to lock a piece of information in a storage unit for later access and use. If I have a satisfying or unsatisfying outcome, it can trigger a like/want/need to repeat it until I know I can do it again. I either want to have the same experience because it felt good, or I want to avoid the same experience because it was not good.
- I think or believe someone else will want me to know this or do this and I want to please them.

- I am practicing something so I can do it better or faster.
- I am doing it over and over because it simply is something to do, which is better than not having anything to do.

Given all this awareness and knowledge, what does it mean for the other person involved in my life when I am repeating things over and over? Whether I am learning something new, trying to hold onto something that is disappearing on me, or trying to repeat something that has given me pleasure or discomfort in the past, you will want to get ready to respond to my repetitions for many reasons:

- Responding allows you to take over control of the direction and intensity of the repetitions, rather than helping to build permanent pathways that result in uncomfortable outcomes or simply take up time.
- Noticing the repetitions and determining their purpose can help guide you in creating alternate pathways to stimulate. The goal is to have a more pleasant outcome for you and me.
- Reacting simply creates more intense or frequent repetitions, since it causes more emotional impact!
- Humans fill time one way or the other. Learning the art of play can change the dynamic of the interaction to one of interest and altered focus, so that you see the

interaction differently, and therefore can alter your side of the interaction for a varied outcome that is satisfactory to both of you.

- You can help others offer a similar and effective pattern of interaction, so that I can get my desired outcome from more people, taking the load off a single responder.

Here is a brief list and description of Five Supportive Communication Strategies to Help Guide Repetitious Questions:

- **Connect** – Use Positive Physical Approach™ (PPA)
- **Reflect** – Provide acknowledgement that the message was received by repeating some of the words
- **Offer** – Give the information being sought in a visual-verbal-physical movement way
- **Interject!** – Pause with a new thought (visually, verbally, and physically) – Signal a lead shift
- **Seek** – Use a Positive Action Starter (PAS) to shift the conversation

These steps will be explained in more detail in another book in this series.

Knowing your person and their agenda, as well as your own, really makes a difference. Where will that person be willing or interested in going in a conversation? What would that person be willing and able to do? What is a go-to activity or place that almost always provides a good feeling or sense of value? What do you want them to do next? Considering all these pieces, how can you get these possibilities to come together?

CHAPTER 12

Motor Skills and Initiation—Let's Get Going!

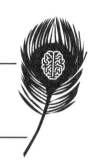

An important concern related to mobility is not particularly well known and can be difficult to see. In the care world, it is referred to as initiation. The ability to get started! It is the act of going from thinking about doing something to actually doing it!

This fairly complex task requires multiple parts of the brain to cooperate in order to get a thought into action. Let's break this ability into the top five elements, to determine where someone still has some function, and where there is a missing ability that will have to be compensated for or supported in a different way.

1. **Desire or will to move** - One piece of the puzzle is whether the person perceives value in moving or doing. Does the person want to move? The desire to move may be to get something of value beyond their

reach or in another location, or it could simply be a desire not to be still any longer.

2. **Comprehension of instructions to begin a movement** - A second piece of the puzzle is whether the person is able to take in auditory information and translate it into a request to do something physically. Is our request enough or the right action step to use first? "Are you thirsty? Let's go get a drink." These questions will only help a person to get going if they can:

   o Understand the information

   o Evaluate their thirst accurately

   o Relate the desire for a drink with the act of getting up

   o Appreciate your willingness to provide them with a drink only if they go with you

3. **Motor initiation** – Once they determine they would like to move or do something, a third element is whether the person can send messages to the motor strip so that action will begin. Can they go from a thinking section of the brain to a movement section of the brain? If not, the person may indicate they do want to do something, but then doesn't get going to do the thing they agreed to do. It is often tricky however, without careful partner work, to figure out if the problem is getting data in, having the person process the request, or having the decision to move be translated into a physical action.

4. **Motor planning or sequencing** – Once initiated, the human brain has to determine what comes next. Each task is broken down into sub-routines, each sub-routine has components. Problems in wiring or storage can cause loss of signals or mis-firings at any point along the way. Hence, we might notice someone leaning forward, but not pushing into a standing position. They might stand in front of a door and not turn the handle to open it or pick up and put down a spoon over and over, but not take a single bite of food.

5. **Distress when starting movement** – If beginning an action causes pain, discomfort, or fear, then immobility and not moving seems to be the better course of action. It is all too easy to assume lack of action is due to dementia, when in fact it might be due to a combination of brain change and arthritis, muscle tenderness, unseen injuries or falls, balance or vestibular issues, vision changes, PTSD, anxiety, or depression.

The first step in changing and getting things going in a better direction is to get curious and try to better understand why things are happening the way they are. Only then can we develop strategies to provide better options, alternatives, and supports.

Take a closer look at these five elements and consider how we could possibly change something to match shifting abilities.

Here's one example to get you going!

If a person doesn't seem to have the desire or will to move in order to redistribute weight, use muscles, or get their needs met, try one of these techniques:

- Will they move automatically to rhythm? If I put on music or if I demonstrate a repetitive action where they can see it, will it cause them to copy me, without the need to understand the value of the action?
- Will they move to music that is from long ago? Rocking lullabies, childhood play music, teenage dance music, or even music to clap to or clap after.
- Is it possible to elicit spontaneous, not thought-about movement? Presenting a non-threating object that can be touched, moved, stroked, or handled. And then moving it slightly further away or providing a second item slightly beyond the first can help a person go from a still state to a moving state.
- Could you use a friendly and alerting sound, plus an action that causes the person to react with action rather than consider whether to move? Say something like, "Teepa, hey! Look at that!" using high energy, a smile, and curiosity in your voice, with a pointing gesture to a high contrast item in the center field of vision.

Keeping someone active and moving is in the best interest of everyone involved. The challenge is figuring out what is getting in the way and what we can choose to do that helps!

CHAPTER 13

Delirium, Depression, and Dementia; Detecting Differences Between the *Three Ds*

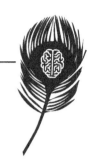

In the medical community the Three Ds are the traditional way of distinguishing changes in cognitive abilities and alterations in mental states or behavioral shifts. It is used by healthcare providers to sort out what is happening and how to address it or fix it. This approach historically pre-supposed that delirium, depression, and dementia were three distinct and unrelated conditions. More recent findings have revealed that they are inter-connected and possibly indicative of the heightened risk for one another.

As people age, their brains become more vulnerable to chemical changes, damage, and disease. Recognizing the differences among changes that signal:

- An acute illness or medical emergency (Delirium)
- Symptoms of a mood or emotional condition (Depression)

- A chronic, progressive, and terminal condition that will eventually rob a person of their cognitive abilities, is vital in providing the best possible care and responding effectively when changes are noted. (Dementia)

Collectively known as the *Three Ds*, delirium, depression, and dementia, each has a unique onset, duration, impact on alertness/arousal, orientation, and possible causes and treatment recommendations. Understanding the differences will allow us to reduce the likelihood of unnecessary hospitalizations, delays in medical attention for acute illness, non-treatment of treatable conditions, and pre-mature discharge of residents in a community setting.

The British Journal of Psychiatry reports[6] that depressed older adults (defined as those over age 50) were more than twice as likely to develop vascular dementia and 65 percent more likely to develop Alzheimers disease than similarly aged people who weren't depressed.

We can't say that late-life depression causes dementia, but we can say it likely contributes to it. We think depression is toxic to the brain, and if you're walking around with some mild brain damage, it will add to the degenerative process.

---

[6] Diniz BS, Butters MA, Albert SM, Dew MA, Reynolds CF 3rd. Late-life depression and risk of vascular dementia and Alzheimer's disease: systematic review and meta-analysis of community-based cohort studies. *Br J Psychiatry*. 2013;202(5):329-335. doi:10.1192/bjp.bp.112.118307

Meryl Butters, an associate professor of psychiatry at the University of Pittsburgh School of Medicine and a co-author of the paper

Episodes of severe delirium have also been linked to an increased risk of dementia. A study[7] conducted by the University of Cambridge and the University of Eastern Finland reports that older people who have experienced episodes of delirium are significantly more likely to develop dementia. There is also strong evidence that people living with dementia have a fifty/fifty chance of showing clinical signs of depression, anxiety, or both. It is vital for all concerned to recognize that as the condition of dementia reaches the late-stages, the destruction of the brain and its ability to guide and coordinate even basic functions of the human body will create an internal environment that causes delirium, and no matter how many times we fix the immediate issue, we cannot fix the dementia, which is what ultimately causes systems to fail. Therefore, learning the art of letting go – not giving up, but letting go – is an essential skill that all care partners and supporters must master to offer best quality care and advocacy.

---

[7] "Delirium Increases the Risk of Developing New Dementia Eight-Fold in Older Patients." *University of Cambridge*, 10 Aug. 2012, www.cam.ac.uk/research/news/delirium-increases-the-risk-of-developing-new-dementia-eight-fold-in-older-patients.

Focusing on Depression

Our brains are wired in such a way that what we think affects both how we feel and what we do. The connections between thinking, feeling, and doing are strong and multi-directional. This means that any one of these features can DRIVE the other two in either a positive or a negative direction. When we have negative thoughts, we feel defeated and don't want to try to do much. It's hard wired in our neurological system. The second consideration is that our systems are most comfortable doing what they routinely do. The more we do something a certain way the more it becomes wired that we will do it that way again, and again, and again. Therefore, if we get into a routine of negative thinking and feeling, we begin to do less and spiral downward into less and less energy and effort, which results in sadness, anger, frustration, inactivity, or negative coping.

So, here is the good news. Working to move in the opposite direction, focusing on positive thinking and feeling, we can reverse the pattern, enabling us to lift ourselves up, and have a positive impact on both delirium and dementia. Building and strengthening new wiring and reinforcing any shift is work and it can be hard. The great news is that once we get the new wiring established and firm it up, it becomes the new routine. As we age, our brains are slower to learn new patterns and new behaviors. It takes longer to build new pathways and to make them the routine. You **can** teach an old dog new tricks, but the trainer needs to be patient, consistent, supportive, and positive!

One caution – depression is both a chemical and a cognitively driven condition. It isn't that the person is **not** trying, it is that the brain chemistry may be making it almost impossible to get the needed energy or sustain the focus without external support and chemical enhancement. This means that **most** depression will need to be treated with a three-part approach:

1. Increased physical activity that provides input to the brain
2. Increased talk therapy that is supportive and provides positive reinforcement inside and out
3. Support (natural and chemical) to help serotonin and dopamine chemistry in the brain become more balanced and effective

Physical strategies that help

- **Determine what to do** – Make a list of physical activities that are doable, repetitive, and use most of the body – get blood flowing, heart pumping, oxygen moving, and lungs working. Examples include: exercise, housework, yard work, car care, laundry, dancing, sweeping, walking, or rolling (if using a wheelchair).
- **Find a partner** – Make of list of people to do the activity with – match talking preferences (if not much of

a talker, limit talking while doing). People who are depressed may find it difficult to get started on their own, so it's critical to create a plan where someone else is involved. Ideally, that someone is a person who can role model, support, connect well with the person, get the action going, and help create a routine.

- **Set a short-term goal and start with baby-steps** – Remember you have to halt the negative and then get out of the inertia, before the positive direction gets going. Start small, then gradually shift up, raising the time limit, the intensity, the frequency, or the repetition a little at a time. Raise the bar so little that the person may not even be aware of it.

Talk therapy

If depression is in the mild to moderate range, talk therapy is likely a good option. The first step is to make sure you find an experienced, qualified therapist, properly trained and credentialed in depression therapy. To find the specific credentials of potential psychotherapists, use the American Psychological Association's (APA) Psychologist Locator, call your local branch of the APA, or ask for a referral from your primary care physician.

What role does dopamine play?[8,9,10]

Dopamine motivates you to take action toward your goals, desires, and needs, and gives you a surge of reinforcing pleasure when achieving them. Procrastination, self-doubt, and lack of enthusiasm are linked with low levels of dopamine.

How can you increase dopamine levels?

Break big goals down into little pieces—rather than only allowing your brain to celebrate when you've hit the finish line, you can create a series of little finish-lines which releases dopamine. And it's crucial to actually celebrate.

What role does serotonin play?

Serotonin flows when you feel significant or important. Loneliness and depression are present when serotonin is absent.

How can you increase serotonin levels?

- Reflecting on past achievements allows your brain to relive the experience. Your brain has trouble telling the

---

[8] "How To Increase Dopamine Levels." *Mental Health Daily*, 29 June 2016, mentalhealthdaily.com/2015/04/17/how-to-increase-dopamine-levels/.
[9] Buckley, Christine. "UConn Researcher: Dopamine Not About Pleasure (Anymore)." *UConn Today*, 10 Dec. 2012, today.uconn.edu/2012/11/uconn-researcher-dopamine-not-about-pleasure-anymore/
[10] McIntosh, James. "Serotonin: Facts, Uses, SSRIs, and Sources." Edited by Debra Rose Wilson, *Medical News Today*, MediLexicon International, 2 Feb. 2018, www.medicalnewstoday.com/articles/232248.php

difference between what's real and imagined, so it produces serotonin in both cases.

- Artificial support to help serotonin and dopamine chemistry: There are also many highly effective ways to increase dopamine levels artificially. Artificial increases in dopamine can be obtained from utilizing pharmaceutical drugs and/or other supplements. While artificial methods for increasing dopamine tend to be the most potent and fastest, most people build up a tolerance to the effect over time. Upon discontinuation of the artificial dopamine booster, most people end up with a dopamine deficiency worse than before they started.

Focusing on Delirium

Delirium is an acute change in abilities that begins rapidly and results in significant shifts in abilities, alertness, arousal, logic, or perceptions. Delirium has a wide array of causes. Some are physiological and physical, while others are emotional, social, or spiritual. If a delirium state is caused by an infection, an electrolyte imbalance, dehydration, sleep deprivation, drug interaction or reaction, an injury, or oxygen deprivation, failure to notice the change or to address what is causing it to happen can and does result in system failure and ultimately death in a short period of time.

There are seven basic elements to consider when trying to

determine whether what is being seen and experienced is more likely related to dementia, depression, or delirium.

Here are seven variables to investigate:

1. **Onset** – When did it start? Was it sudden, recent, or more gradual?

2. **Duration** – How long has it been going on and do the symptoms seem to be stable or on/off? Present unless the condition is fixed, present unless the condition is addressed, worsening over time until death?

3. **Alertness and Arousal** – How awake and attentive is the person? Does it fluctuate from hyper- to hypo-arousal and alertness, not change from baseline that much, gradually get more and more problematic?

4. **Orientation Responses** – How able is the person to be aware of place, time, person, and situation? Is it highly variable from one hour to the next? Are phrases such as "I don't know" or "It doesn't matter" common? Do they give inaccurate but related answers or ask why you need to know?

5. **Mood and Affect** – What is the emotional state and variability of the person? Are they highly variable, depending on their physical condition? Are they flat, angry, sad, laughing, or giddy without cause, or negative? Are they triggered by what is happening around them, or changing over time?

6. **Possible Causes** – What is triggering or causing these

changes? Is it more physiological or acute emotional distress? Is it seasonal, chemical, or situational? Is it due to brain chemistry and structural changes that are progressing?

7. **Treatment Impact** – What treatments might be more helpful? Identify the source of the change and remediate it. Use a combination of the right mood or psychiatric medication, talk therapy, and activity to resolve or manage symptoms. Use supportive approaches and environmental modifications, with possibly considering medications to support and help with function, since there are still no known cures or medications that slow or halt dementia.

Why is it so important that family members and care providers are familiar with these different conditions? Due to the possibility that all three can be present in one individual and that the treatments vary widely, it is vital that someone who knows the person's baseline abilities is part of the assessment of any situation that arises. This is essential as the person's ability to represent themselves and their perception is so significantly altered by any of the three, and without additional guidance, assumptions about baseline abilities can have unintended consequences or changes in ability can be missed or misunderstood. Having a knowledgeable and capable advocate can make a huge difference in what is done if a person experiences a sudden change in abilities with an underlying very minimal impairment state. If someone has Lewy Body Disease, however, it is essential that they are not mistaken for having schizophrenia and having their symptoms misman- aged with anti-psychotics which are considered high-risk medications for the dementia condition.[11,12]

In summary, here is a visual that shows how these different conditions relate. As you think about the conditions of delir- ium, depression, anxiety, and dementia relate, remember:

- They can look similar
- They frequently happen to the same person
- Some are fixable, some are not
- People with dementia can have all of them
- People with dementia can have all of them happening at the same time or at different times
- They have different causes and consequences!

In the next chapter, we will discuss how to determine the right type of health support for dementia.

---

[11] Source: Graham, Judith. "Does Depression Contribute to Dementia?" The New Old Age Blog. The New York Times, 1 May 2013. Web. 11 Apr. 2016. http://newoldage.blogs.nytimes.com/2013/05/01/does- depression-contribute-to-dementia/?_r=0

[12] http://www.cam.ac.uk/research/news/delirium-increases-the-risk-of-developing-new- dementia-eight-fold-in-older-patients, 12 Aug.2010. http://creativecommons.org/licenses/by-nc-sa/3.0/

How Delirium, Depression, Anxiety, and Dementia Relate

Anxiety
Signals an upward spiral that is treatable.

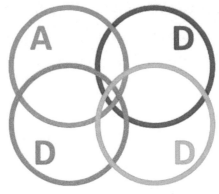

Dementia
Signals a change in abilities that does progress, cannot be halted or cured, will vary by disease type, and *yet* progression is highly dependent on environmental support, social support, and personal decisions.

Delirium
Signals an acute change in abilities that fluctuate. Check it out!

Depression
Signals a downward spiral that is treatable.

Graphic 15

Please use this QR code for a more detailed look at how all three conditions relate, including the symptoms and triggers for each.

Scan this code with your smartphone's camera or visit **www.teepasnow.com/moreinfo** on your computer.

CHAPTER 14

What Next? Five Types of Health Support for People Living with Dementia

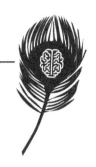

We typically do NOT spend a lot of time considering which form of health care we should be seeking when we are healthy and well. If we were to get acutely ill, of course, we would get ourselves treated. When we are well, we typically want to reduce our risks of getting a chronic disease or hastening the onset of possible health problems. However, we rarely follow through on doing *all* that we can to reduce those risks; it is too much trouble, too costly, too extreme, or even too poorly researched to justify the value. In other words, it seems like too much work for the possibility of benefits. As part of our lack of attention to this situation, we do NOT complete our advance directives and discuss them with the person we think will be our durable health care power of attorney (our surrogate decision maker) when we are well and whole. And even if we do a bit of that, we keep it general and really don't look seriously about our genetic codes and life-style risks. So how does this relate to receiving a diagnosis of dementia?

Let's think about five possible approaches to health care:

1. **Preventive** – keep something from happening
2. **Curative** – get something to stop happening and then return to a previous level of function and health
3. **Restorative** – regain some abilities or learn to do things a new way after an event/episode/illness that changed abilities, through the use of rehabilitation and compensatory strategies
4. **Maintenance** – keep something from getting worse, when getting better is not really an option
5. **Palliative** – provide support and comfort as the condition or illness is progressing

Each of these is unique in its focus and techniques to be used. Each has a role and place in our care and well-being, but no one single approach can really meet our needs throughout our life and throughout the course of any long-term illness.

If some form of dementia presents itself, everything we think and know about *what* we should be doing and *who* should be doing it will be called into question. Suddenly, we may become hyper-vigilant or aggressive in our approaches. We can turn into zealots or brutal task masters in our efforts to not leave any stone unturned and to do all that we can do to try to help. Some healthcare providers, when relaying that the diagnosis is dementia, immediately jump into late-stage care considerations even though the person is still in the early-stages of the condition. Rarely, do we step back and consider the range of health care alternatives. Rarer still is our interest in thinking the options through carefully to determine what makes sense at any point in time and to plan for the proba-bilities of the future.

Use this QR code to view a support table that explores these five healthcare options in more detail.

Scan this code with your smartphone's camera or visit **www.teepasnow.com/moreinfo** on your computer.

Each is unique and has a place in our lives. The question is complex, but which one is the right one for you and the per-son you are supporting, at which stages of change, and how will you know that?

I have provided a few resources that are available to help you begin to explore what you might want to consider **first** for yourself, and **then** with the person living with dementia. Some of the resources have been posted by people living with dementia and they represent their perspective and point of view. Others are provided by agencies or organizations devoted to helping people retain control over their lives as they change due to an acute event, a chronic or progressive illness, or a terminal condition. Since dementia involves all these situations, it gets complicated. It is crucial to talk about it **before** it becomes a crisis or surprises us. Take the time to consider what you think and want before you enter the emotionally charged atmosphere of a hospital emergency room, a doctor's office, a rehabilitation center, a nursing home, an assisted living community, memory care, or hospice support. Advanced planning allows us time to work through options rather than *choose* by default without considering the past, present, and future for the person and ourselves.

Let's consider whether the choice is really what our partner would want, because that makes a difference. Perhaps there is an opportunity to pull the team together and talk it through. Having a conversation about what is possible can ultimately empower us to determine the best course of action, given the full picture of where we have been, where we are, and where we are headed. The good thing about thinking ahead is there will be time to reconsider as things change.

There are many resources available to support your preferences and intentions for care. Resources such as these are vital to living a better quality life and being intentional about your choices. Here are just a few:

Additional Resources:

- Five Wishes – This organization provides an advance directive document which helps people discuss and document their wishes in a non-threatening, life-affirming way. https://fivewishes.org/
- *Providing Comfort Care to People with Dementia During Their Last Days of Life – A guide for family and friends –* Northern Ireland Version
- https://research.hscni.net/sites/default/files/Comfort Care Booklet.pdf
- *Forget me not: palliative care for people with dementia* by Dr. Dylan Harris. A post-graduate article discussing the role of palliative care in dementia.
- https://www.ncbi.nlm.nih.gov/pmc/articles/PMC2600060/

CHAPTER 15

Teepa and Her Team
Answer Your Questions

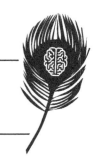

This book, and the series it is starting, tries to help bring awareness to life with dementia – how it affects the person living with the condition and the others around that person. In addition to the articles included in this book, we wanted to address some questions that we often get regarding dementia.

Teepa wanted the team to provide answers, while she offered additional ideas or insights. Take a look at the questions below and our responses. Let us know if you have other questions you'd like to see answered, by using our website posting option.

Scan this code with your smartphone's camera or visit **www.teepasnow.com/moreinfo** on your computer.

Two different questions about the temporal lobe changes that are typically part of dementia:

1. Is it true people always keep music, poetry, prayer, and counting?
2. Why is it that people who get dementia use foul or unacceptable language when they never did it before they got the condition?

Teepa's Response:

1. There is rarely an *always* in the world of dementia. It is certainly very, very common for there to be a retention of rhythm related skills when someone develops dementia. It is not until late in most dementias that rhythm abilities are more severely impacted, compared to skilled and thought-related abilities. If people learned songs, dances, rhythm based actions or phrases when they were younger, it is very likely they will be able to access and use these patterns well into their condition. Unfortunately, language comprehension, vocabulary, and speech production are much more likely to be lost earlier on. Keeping these abilities may also be related to their role in survival. These rhythmic patterns can both soothe, calm, and comfort as well as excite and stimulate, depending on how they are used. It's a good thing to think about both, because rest and action are both essential to life.

2. There is a big difference between knowing foul and inappropriate words, and using them when our brains are mature and working effectively. The combination of reduced impulse control, loss of vocabulary options, and more intense sense of threat or discomfort can supply the basic answer to this question. It's not that I want to use those words or phrases, it is that those are the words that are still available, I may be feeling distressed or am seeking to share something, and I can't access my alternatives or control the impulse.

Dan's and Debi's response:

Dementia doesn't give us too many gifts, but rhythm tends to be one of them. In Chapter 6 *Do You Hear What I Say?*, Teepa talked about the changes in the left temporal lobe. With the changes there, people living with dementia tend to lose vocabulary, comprehension, and speech production. However, the right temporal lobe is often less affected by dementia. So what is stored over there?

- Social chit-chat – the idea that I talk, you talk, I talk, you talk
- Rhythm of speech – how a question goes up at the end, tone of voice
- Rhythm in language– found in music, poetry, prayer, counting, and spelling

- The connection to automatic rhythmic movements like humming, clapping, swaying or rocking, and even dancing
- Forbidden words – sex talk, racial slurs, mean or degrading words and phrases
  - These words were stored in a different place than the regular vocabulary because they held an emotional component and were socially unacceptable

So what does this mean for a person supporting a person living with dementia? You now have tools to connect with those who aren't able to participate in a conversation like they once were:

- A person who isn't able to form a full sentence can sing a song from their teenage years or say familiar prayers
- Clapping, rocking side to side, and dancing together can be a wonderful connector
- When the synapses in the brain fire like this, you see that other connections in the brain are found, even for a brief moment.
- When we let go of what was and learn to appreciate the gifts of what we have now, it will allow us all to find joy and connection together.

Wait a minute, did you mean to say forbidden language was a gift, too?

Yes, actually we did. We know that seems a bit odd, and it can certainly lead to some awkward moments, but let's take a closer look. The first thing we need to do is train ourselves to respond to these words instead of react. We also need to look past the words to understand the situation as well as the tone, volume, and intensity of their words.

- For our first example, let's say we heard someone in a restaurant ask in a curious way, but loud enough for many to hear, "What's that big, fat guy eating over there? That looks good."

First, we need to take a deep breath and listen to the tone. Was it said in a malicious or mean way? In this case, it seems to be general curiosity. So why choose those words? Well, the brain is used to going to the temporal lobes to find the words they want. When the left temporal lobe is struggling and unable to provide the socially acceptable words, the brain goes to the right temporal lobe. It found words over there to help get the message across, so the brain chose those. If this is the case, here are our two choices –

1. Ask in an equally curious tone, "you're wanting to know what the man in the red sweater is eating? Mmm, that does look good."

2. Correct them with a sharp, warning tone, "We don't say things like that. My goodness!"

Which of these is more likely to be our first reaction? Which of these is more likely to provide a better outcome?

- In our second example, let's say I'm trying to help someone change pants after an incontinence episode. The woman screams "Stop, stop you stupid, ugly whore! Help!"

Was this said in the same curious tone as in the first example? No, definitely not. The volume, tone, and intensity are very high, even though I am just trying to help. Instead of blaming her, I need to look at how I set up the situation. Was she aware of why I was wanting to help? Did she give me permission? Or, from her perspective, was I trying to take off her pants, possibly in front of others? Could I have triggered a traumatic memory from her past?

In this case, she is using those forbidden words as her last line of verbal defense as she feels she is being attacked. Again, here are two options to choose from:
1. Yell back "I'm just trying to help!"
2. Step back, take a deep breath and say sincerely, "I am so sorry, I was trying to help. That shouldn't have happened."

Which of these is likely to be our first reaction? We were trying to help, after all. However, did we work to connect with her, get her permission, and do the task with her?

Using what remains in the right temporal lobe can be a gift to help us connect with, and understand, people living with dementia. We will need to use our best efforts to take a deep breath and respond versus allowing our amygdala to react.

Is a specific diagnosis important? Aren't all dementias basically the same?

Dan's and Debi's Response

Did you know that there are over 120 different types, forms, and causes of dementia? (Teepa's note: that I have identified at least. I base this estimate on years of clinical and academic practice. It is interesting to note, however, that little has been done to actually classify or intensely study this complex world until very recently.)

For any of these 120+ types, forms, and causes to be considered a dementia, there are four truths that need to apply:

- At least two parts of the brain are dying
- It is progressive and will get worse
- It is chronic – there is no cure or treatment
- It is fatal

So, if at least two parts of the brain are dying, that leads to many combinations that can be affected. On top of that, there are areas within each of those sections that will be affected differently. For instance, with Alzheimers you will probably notice memory loss earlier in the condition, but with Frontotemporal Dementia, memory loss won't be noticeable until the disease progresses much further. Lewy Body Dementia can often come with hallucinations, but when an anti-psychotic medicine is used to combat the hallucinations, it can prove dangerous or fatal. Vascular dementia is very dependent on the physical health, diet, and exercise of the person living with dementia. With some types of dementias, a person may only live for six more months, while with other types, a person may live another 30 years.

Teepa has given us tips and taught us skills that will work with all forms of dementia people are living with, but each type will require different care and support. The more we know with a specific diagnosis, the better position we can put ourselves in to succeed.

What does dementia have to do with vision?

Teepa's response:

Vision is one of the primary ways we get data from the world around us into our brain. It is also critical in using our bodies to interact with that world. Visual processing is controlled in large part by the brain. There are many aspects to vision that are going to be affected by various forms of dementia, but one that is almost universal is that the amount of data you can take in and process at any moment in time will be more limited. That means I can either scan a large area and actually *see* very little, or keep my eyes focused on a smaller area and see less of the larger world. The area that I can take in at one time is referred to as my visual field. Other vision related skills that change with dementia include organized scanning, object recognition, depth perception, figure-ground awareness, color perception, and tracking, just to name a few.

Dan's and Debi's response:

What does dementia have to do with vision? Quite a lot, actually. In Chapter 7, Teepa discussed *Changing Our Visual Awareness* in which she talked about the physical components of vision as well as the different types of vision we have. In that section she also talked about Targeted Vision, Central Field Vision, Peripheral Vision, and Far Peripheral Vision. Let's look at how age and dementia affect those four areas.

Once we hit about 25 years of age, our brains start to slow down. This isn't dementia, this is normal aging. As our brain slows, it simply can't process as much information as quickly as it once could. As Teepa mentioned, vision is our favorite way to accept incoming data, so what do we do with it all? The brain prioritizes what it feels is most important, which would be our Targeted and Central Field Vision. That leaves our Far Peripheral Vision, so we start to lose a few degrees each year, but it happens so slowly we don't tend to notice it.

However, as we get closer to 75 years old instead of 25 years old, we realize as we're driving that we need to turn our heads a bit more to make sure that blind spot is clear. As we get to 75 and beyond, turning our heads may not be enough, we may have to turn our shoulders and then our car follows us, too! Maybe it is time for a defensive driving course, some flexibility exercises, or at least a check on self-awareness related to abilities in this area, to reduce risks in motor vehicles.

If that is normal aging, what happens when dementia is present?

- Please remember, when talking about vision changing with dementia, it doesn't mean that the eyes aren't working. The brain simply can't process all of the data, so it prioritizes what it feels is most important.

- I'm going to do my best to describe what happens, but I'd like you to try some things, too. Please use Graphic 12 titled *Visual Cortex* found at the end of Chapter 7 as a guide.

In the **early-stages** of dementia, a person's active field of vision is similar to what they might experience if they were wearing a scuba mask.

- Try this – put your hands around your eyes with your fingers touching above your eyes and your thumbs touching each side of your nose, below your eyes. Look around to notice what you can see and what you can't see.

As dementia progresses to the **mid-stages**, visual field changes even more to what we refer to as binocular vision.

- Try this – put your hands around your eyes as if you were wearing binoculars. Have your thumbs meet the fingers of the same hand around your eyes. Look around again, what can you see and what can't you see? If you had a stain on your shirt, could you see it? If you are in a safe place, try walking around and notice what you have to do to navigate the environment.

Still in the **mid-stages**, but with the dementia progressing a bit more, a person will retain binocular vision, but will start to lose object recognition. This means they'll see an object, possibly recognize it, but not know what to do with it.

- Think about it this way – at a table they may pick up a fork, but not use it to move the food from the plate to their mouth. In the bathroom, they may see a hair brush and a toothbrush both near the toothpaste, but not know which one to use. They both have handles and bristles, after all.

Moving to the **late-stages** of dementia, the brain is struggling to keep up even more and is only able to process the information from one eye.

- Try this – close one eye and use one hand around the open eye. Reach out to something in front of you, with the hand that is not around your eye, to see if you can tell when your fingers will touch it. With monocular vision, not only is our field smaller, but we lose depth perception. This can lead to falls or fear of movement as I try to reach down to pick up something that I think is closer than it is.

In the **final stage** of dementia, a person's brain is working hard just to keep their internal processes moving. A person won't be able to have their eyes open much or for very long. They will have a very limited visual field when their eyes are open, so using touch and verbal cues will be important.

Vision plays an incredibly important role in our lives, so we need to be aware of what the other person is able to see and how they interact with what is in their visual field.

Why do People Living with Dementia always say "I want to go home" when they are already where they live?

Teepa's response:

It is very rare that someone will *always* say this. Typically, I find it comes up at certain times and in some patterned ways.

When someone says this, it usually means that they are seeking another place, time, person, or situation. It is an indicator of brain change in the hippocampal area combined with a primitive desire to seek that which the person believes will provide the essentials for survival and well-being. It should be a signal to those around that some sort of change is needed, or at least an assessment of stress-distress level is indicated. It can be an indicator of an unmet human need of some sort.

Dan's and Debi's response:

To answer this question, we have to think about what home is. Is it a structure with walls and a ceiling? Sure. Is our home more than that? To many people, it definitely is. Home is where the heart is, after all.

What does the idea of home mean to many of us? A place of familiarity, safety, and love. It is also a place of feeling accepted, supported, and where mistakes are forgiven.

When someone tells you they want to go home, even when they are where they currently live, they are often saying that something doesn't feel right. Teepa likes to describe a place using the four Fs:

1. Friendly
2. Familiar
3. Functional
4. Forgiving

When a person doesn't feel comfortable somewhere, it is often because the space is lacking in one or more of the four Fs. Something doesn't feel right and they want to go somewhere that does feel right. The place of sanctuary that many of us have returned to over the years is *home*.

One thing to try might be to reflect their words back to them in a tone of voice similar to theirs.

I've heard People Living with Dementia will start behaving badly and turn aggressive, is that true?

Teepa's response:

From my perspective there are several concerns that come from this sort of statement. First, it seems to separate People Living with Dementia into a group of them versus us. I am pretty sure there are people in this world who have never and will never become aggressive or behave badly in the eyes of at least one other person. I am also fairly certain that I have both behaved badly and been aggressive, according to myself and others, and it is certainly not due to any dementia. Part of my world view is that we all have the potential to feel overwhelmed and threatened in certain situations.

Some of these situations are predictable and some of them are not. When we find ourselves in those conditions, if we have a healthy and mature brain, we may or may not be able to control our primitive survival reaction and instead use our executive control center, our thinking brain, to resolve it.

As far as which primitive survival strategy our brain picks, it really depends on our past, the situation, and our sense of danger. Should I flight, fight, hide, or seek? We have personal patterns. Typically, dementia will strip away our ability to respond and leaves us with our reactions. So what happens around, and to, the Person Living with Dementia, combined with both the person's history and life patterns, and the type and degree of dementia, will all be factors in how they react.

Dan's and Debi's response:

First let's take a look at the words that we are using to describe what's happening. Words like aggressive, resistant, and behaviors indicate blame, that someone is at fault, or that someone is choosing to be difficult. What is actually happening is that we both find ourselves in a challenging situation. Sometimes pausing and taking a step back to see the big picture and the people involved can help us reach a more productive and positive interaction for everyone.

Here is a list of some examples that can cause anyone, whether they are living with dementia or not, to react in a way that appears to be irritable, defensive, or aggressive:

- Having an unmet physical or emotional need
- Being startled

- Having something done to you that you didn't understand or agree to
- Trying to express yourself and people can't understand you
- Feeling judged by others

Think about how you have felt when experiencing any of the items on the list above, or maybe even more than one at a time. Are you always able to respond with the same level of kindness and understanding that you have when you are comfortable, and all of your needs have been met? For most of us, the answer is no – and we have healthy brains!

If you remember in Chapter 5 when Teepa talked about the primitive brain versus the thinking brain, as dementia progresses, the amygdala (threat perceiver) can go on higher alert. This can make things seem threatening even when they weren't meant to be. Dementia doesn't cause aggression, so when we see these challenging situations, we need to take on the role of a detective and figure out what happened, what led up to that moment. Then, just as importantly, what can we do differently next time to help lead to a better interaction for us all.

Something to keep in mind is to track when these challenging situations occur. Do they tend to happen at the same time each day? What about location, do they tend to occur in the same part of the house? Maybe it's a particular task – such as eating/drinking, dressing/undressing, bathing, or toileting. When we start to notice patterns, we can adapt and try something different.

When we step back and take a deep breath, we can recognize that all of us, including People Living with Dementia are doing the best we can in any given moment.

Why do People Living with Dementia keep telling the same stories or ask the same questions over and over?

Teepa's response:

They want to get connected and they are using familiar phrases, memories, and patterns of interaction to do so, or they want to find out something about what is happening and they are seeking help from a trusted source. In both situations, it is a seeking behavior. Finding ways to respond and then transition to an alternative activity, place, or situation can be a skill worth developing.

Dan's and Debi's response:

That's a great question, but I feel like I've heard it before.

Repetition of stories or questions generally boils down to one of two things; anxiety, or wanting a connection. The hippocampus in the brain is in charge of learning and remembering, wayfinding, and the passage of time. When that is damaged, it is really difficult to hold on to new information. If a person living with dementia asks you a question like "What time is my appointment?" or "What are we having for dinner?" and no matter how many times you answer, they still come back and ask again, it is probably due to damage in the hippocampus. They are trying to put that information into a storage cabinet in their brain that just isn't working the way it once was. Not only that, they may not remember that they asked, so they ask again.

As for the telling of stories, why do any of us like to tell stories, jokes, or interesting anecdotes? We get to share something with someone else, hopefully bring them joy, and become connected with them. With damage to that hippocampus mentioned a moment ago, a person living with dementia can't remember that they already told you, so it's new for them. It can be annoying or even frustrating to hear it over and over, but we recommend learning that story. When the disease progresses further and they aren't able to tell the story, you can start the story or even tell the whole thing. This will help build your connection throughout the journey.

Epilogue

Now that you have completed this book, what are your thoughts? What are you feeling and thinking about what is happening for you and the people around you? How does what you have taken in change or support the life you are living? Have you discovered anything that might guide or direct you toward a better pathway as you continue onward?

In closing, take a look at these two sponges. Then imagine them as two brains: one that is healthy and one that has been living with dementia for a long time. (Brains shrink when dementia advances.)

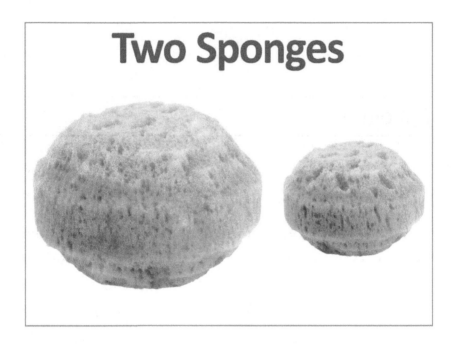

Graphic 16

Which sponge one can hold more water?

The larger one, most probably.

Which *brain* might be able to better handle stress?

Probably the larger and more complete and complex one.

Which brain might be helpful?

Well, I suspect that would depend on what you were doing with it.

Which might be more interesting to have in your life?

To me, that depends on what I am interested in at any time, what is happening in my life.

Is there value in each?

Absolutely, each brain and sponge has value and purpose. Why judge the value of one over the other, when it is possible that each has something unique and valuable to offer.

Is it possible to have moments of pleasure in engaging with either brain?

It really depends on where I am and what I am capable of enjoying.

Why am I showing you these two sponges? Because, if you have read this book, you might not have been able to take in everything that was in it all at once. You might, however, find value in taking in smaller amounts with a focus on what you are trying to do or trying to understand at any one time.

If you are looking for something more to fill you up, then consider checking out some other support resources or options.

Most of all, celebrate the idea that each of us has purpose and value when we are willing to find the place and space we are designed to fill!

About the Author

An Occupational Therapist by profession, Teepa Snow graduated from Duke University and has an MS degree from the University of North Carolina in Chapel Hill. She has worked in a wide variety of settings and taught at the university level. Teepa works closely with clinical researchers in geriatrics and has extensive experience in neurological care settings. She has dedicated over four decades to her mission of improving dementia care, impacting hundreds of organizations worldwide with her training, books, and DVDs, now sold in over 30 countries. It is through this rich and diverse career, filled with opportunities and challenges, that Teepa has become recognized and sought after as a leader in dementia care.

Teepa founded Positive Approach, LLC in 2007 with the mission of changing the culture of dementia care, one mind at a time. While it started as a one woman show, Positive Approach, LLC, is now an international dementia care training, educational, and consulting organization which helps healthcare professionals and families transform what exists into a more positive dementia care culture.

Until There's A Cure, There's Care™

Made in the USA
Coppell, TX
01 March 2023